Comp Therapy.

Doctors Talking with Patients/Patients Talking with Doctors

Doctors Talking with Patients/Patients Talking with Doctors

IMPROVING COMMUNICATION IN MEDICAL VISITS

DEBRA L. ROTER & JUDITH A. HALL

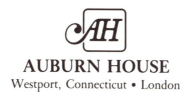

AUBURN HOUSE

Westport, Connecticut • London

Library of Congress Cataloging-in-Publication Data

Roter, Debra.
    Doctors talking with patients/patients talking with doctors :
improving communication in medical visits / Debra L. Roter & Judith
A. Hall.
       p.   cm.
    Includes bibliographical references and index.
    ISBN 0–86569–048–0 (alk. paper)
    1. Physician and patient. 2. Communication in medicine.
I. Hall, Judith A. II. Title.
    [DNLM: 1. Communication. 2. Office Visits. 3. Physician-Patient
Relations. W 62 R843d]
R727.3.R68 1992
610.69′6—dc20   92–17633
DNLM/DLC
for Library of Congress

British Library Cataloguing in Publication Data is available.

Library of Congress Catalog Card Number: 92–17633
ISBN: 0–86569–048–0

First published in 1992

Auburn House, 88 Post Road West, Westport, CT 06881
An imprint of Greenwood Publishing Group, Inc.

Printed in the United States of America

The paper used in this book complies with the
Permanent Paper Standard issued by the National
Information Standards Organization (Z39.48-1984).

10 9 8 7 6 5 4 3 2 1

Copyright Acknowledgment

Excerpts reproduced, with permission, from A.L. Suchman and D.A. Matthews, What makes the
patient-doctor relationship therapeutic?: Exploring the connexional dimension of medical care. *Annals
of Internal Medicine*. 1988; vol. 108: 125–130.

Contents

Tables

Preface

There are important ways in which the exchanges of doctors and patients can be improved, for the benefit of both. In emphasizing the doctor-patient relationship, we do not imply, however, that all the woes of the medical system can be traced to that source. In the United States, ever-rising costs of health care are a terrible burden to the economy, and millions of citizens cannot get or afford proper medical care. This dilemma, just one of many, is not solved by studying what happens within the four walls of a doctor's office.

But what happens within those walls is extremely important—the words and gestures, the decisions, the attitudes, and the presumptions held on both sides are key elements of the medical experience. Encounters with doctors are highly charged—often comforting and rewarding, sometimes upsetting and disappointing. Not only do people remember, often word for word, some exchange with a doctor, but these exchanges are frequently recited for family members and friends. For some people, the words of the remembered dialogue during a past medical visit in themselves take on the full significance of a life event, creating distress anew in each repetition—or providing comfort and reassurance.

The significance of doctor-patient communication goes far beyond personal hopes and disappointments, for years of research now proves that these exchanges have far-reaching impact. A patient's interest in the health care process, willingness to visit doctors, cooperativeness, knowledge, and health itself can be traced to the character of these exchanges.

Like many who study health and illness and the process of medical care, we believe that medical care is a social process as well as a technical one. In other words, medical care involves more than correct diagnosis and recommendation of treatment. Social factors precede diagnosis, for they are involved in the very experience and definition of illness and the willingness to seek care. Social and psychological processes imbue every event and decision in medical care. Medicine is not a narrowly defined technical enterprise, no matter how sophisticated the technologies become. Many doctors and patients undoubtedly recognize how profoundly social the process of medical care is, but probably few, in either group, are aware of how well developed our scientific knowledge of that process is.

In writing this book, we hope to introduce this important body of research to those who will profit from it most—the doctors and patients who have been its subject.

The book is not an attack on doctors, any more than it is an attack on patients. Doctors and patients share the responsibility for shortcomings in their relationships, and together they can work to correct them. If we take it as our job to communicate these shortcomings, we do so in the hope of enhancing the medical experience for both.

Our focus in writing this book is, as the title suggests, talk. The term *talk* is meant broadly, to include all of the face-to-face communications, including nonverbal, that are exchanged between doctors and patients. We use the vernacular word *doctor* to refer to a person with an M.D. or D.O. degree. The word *physician* is interchangeable. We sometimes also refer to providers and practitioners, terms that include doctors along with other professionals who provide health care, such as nurses, nurse practitioners, and physicians' assistants.

Underlying the work presented in this book is the confidence that doctors and patients can change the nature of their interactions. If we accomplish nothing else, we hope to encourage doctors and patients to reflect on the possibility of eliciting new repertoires of response from one another. This requires gaining insight into how each typically behaves, developing an agenda for what an improved relationship would look like, and recognizing that a person tends to act consistently with the other's expectations. Our goal is to convey enough knowledge to convince doctors and patients of the necessity for change, and to promote a sense of empowerment in them. We do this in what we hope is a logical manner, drawing on findings from our own research and that of others.

STRUCTURE OF THE BOOK

The book is divided into four parts. Part I is descriptive in nature and designed to reflect what is known about how doctors and patients typically behave from a variety of vantage points.

The first chapter presents a broad overview of the significance of talk to the doctor-patient relationship and the therapeutic process. The significance of talk is discussed within the context of seven communication-enhancing principles designed to demonstrate not only the critical role talk plays in the medical care process, but that the talk of the visit can be changed for the better. Moreover, the implications of transformed talk are pivotal to the fundamental way medicine is practiced. It is the first step to a transformed medical model that is patient-centered and optimally effective.

The second chapter explores the form of the doctor-patient relationship. The variety of relationship models presented explores the unstated ground rules for routine exchanges and provides insight into the rich diversity of forms that relationships may take. These forms range from strong authority and paternalism to collaborative partnerships, with much variation in between. The focus of the chapter is the varying nature of talk, which, during the medical visit, supports and molds the form the relationship will take.

There are a variety of factors that contribute to how a doctor or patient may behave during the medical visit. Some of these factors are highly individual, such as personality traits and prior experience—but many factors are not. Sociodemographic characteristics, for instance, are quite predictive of both patient and physician behavior. The third and fourth chapters of the book address both social and personal characteristics affecting patient and provider behavior. For patients, a rich literature is reviewed documenting the important influence on talk of such sociodemographic variables as age, race, gender, education, and social class. The effect of such things as physical appearance and likability is not nearly as well documented, but appears also to be important.

The literature is less rich in the description of physician characteristics associated with visit talk and the care given to patients. Nonetheless, physician gender appears to affect the length of a medical visit, the content emphasis, and to some extent the treatment a patient is likely to experience during the visit. Other physician characteristics, such as job satisfaction and attitudes toward the psychological component of medical problems, may also be associated with the care given.

Part II of the book presents a snapshot of routine medical visits. This bird's-eye view is intended to provide the reader with a sense of script and insight into how predictable the structure and talk of the medical visit really are. In Chapter 5 we offer an analysis of the dialogue of doctors and patients. We describe how medical visits proceed and what doctors and patients typically talk about. The information here should be both familiar—readers will no doubt recognize aspects of the visits they have had—and surprising in the realization of how standardized most exchanges are.

Not all talk is equally important to the care process. Two categories of talk are particularly critical. The first is information exchange and the second is talk in the emotional realm. While on the surface these aspects of talk appear to be quite different, they in fact share many functions in the care process. Chapter 6 describes the two-way flow of information in encounters and its role in determining authority and dominance, as well as in substantively providing the basis for mutual understanding between physician and patient.

Part III goes beyond the typical to discuss the range of variation that is evident in the behavior of doctors and patients, and what some of the causes and consequences of that variation might be. Chapter 7 describes variation in the technical quality of medical care, and how differences in talk relate to variation in quality of care.

A shift from possible antecedents to consequences of care is made in Chapter 8, in which patient satisfaction with care, compliance with medical recommendations, functional status, quality of life, and morbidity are traced to variations in the nature of medical visit talk. Chapter 9 demonstrates the surprising ease with which important improvements in the process and outcome of care can be achieved through experimental interventions.

Finally, in Part IV, we speculate on the nature of doctor-patient relations in the future.

Acknowledgments

A number of wonderful people have helped by giving us ideas and criticizing drafts of chapters. These include Fred Gordon, Nancy Hall, Ed Krupat, Mark Knapp, and Rima Rudd. We wish particularly to thank physician friends who not only criticized drafts but helped sensitize us to the physician's point of view as a reader: Arnold Epstein, R. Heather Palmer, Klea Bertakis, Timothy Quill, and Mack Lipkin, Jr. Susan Waller did much to sensitize us to the patient's point of view. Susan Larson, our valued colleague, helped immeasurably in the preparation of this book and the conduct of much of our research. We extend warm thanks to Max Hall, whose advice on writing style was taken over and over.

We are especially grateful to John Harney, our editor, who encouraged and supported us, making timely publication of this book possible.

The most meaningful support in the writing of this book has come from our spouses, Eric Waller and Fred Gordon. And, of course, from our children: Saul, Benjamin, and Annie Rose, and Jacob, Rebecca, and Sarah.

Finally, we thank each other—for making up for each other's defects, for inspiration, and for being there for one another.

Part I

The Nature of the Doctor-Patient Relationship

1

The Significance of Talk

This book is about doctors and patients and what goes on between them in medical visits. Most of what occurs is talk. By talk we mean what is said in the usual sense—the words that are used, the facts exchanged, the advice given, and the social amenities that tie the conversation together. But we also mean communication beyond words, the whole repertoire of nonverbal expressions and cues. The smiles and head nods of recognition, the grimaces of pain, the high-pitched voice of anxiety all give context and enhanced meaning to the words spoken. Despite its central role, for the most part this talk goes unnoticed. There are exceptions: a doctor pays deliberate attention to which questions to ask, and might take conscious note of a look of perplexity on the patient's face. A patient may phrase a question ahead of time or lament oversights in the description of symptoms. But generally the exchange is taken for granted, and participants have little sense that they choose how it develops or that it can be different than it typically is.

The perspective of this book is that talk is the main ingredient in medical care and that it is the fundamental instrument by which the doctor-patient relationship is crafted and by which therapeutic goals are achieved. Though physicians conduct physical exams and use blood tests, X-rays, medications, and much else to achieve therapeutic goals, the value of these activities is limited without the talk that organizes the history and symptoms and puts them in a meaningful context for both patients and physicians.

Our high regard for the role of talk is far from universally accepted. Historians of modern medicine have tracked the changing patterns of medical practice to reveal a fundamental shift in the centrality of talk to the care process. In his study of the history of doctors and patients, Edward Shorter (1985) identifies the post–World War II era as a pivotal time for modern medicine. The discovery of sulfa drugs in the 1930s and later penicillin in the 1940s transformed the practice of medicine. The transformation was, however, not so much in the prescription of these drugs but in their impact on medical training. The drug revolution led medicine to the chemistry-oriented sciences of biochemistry, microbiology, pharmacology, immunology, and genetics and a mainly organic picture of disease to be combated with drugs. The battlelines were drawn between the doctor and the aberrant molecules, with the patient often left on the sidelines. Hence the birth of the biomedical model of disease and medicine's diminished interest in the patient's experience of illness.

Shorter maintains that the practical fact of this depersonalization of medicine was the downgrading in importance of taking the patient's history and giving a physical exam in lieu of more structured data collection and interpretation of laboratory data. It is not coincidental that the practice of interviewing patients using a written outline designed around a series of yes-no questions began during this time. Patient talk was largely curtailed by these changes; patients were restricted to answering the questions asked. One important effect of these changes was to recast medical dialogue as wholly scientific and objective with a goal of keeping patient emotion in check.

In some part, the focus on scientific objectivity reflects a widespread characterization of medicine as taking place in a context of potential death, disability, trauma, pain, and uncertainty. Patients are thought to defend themselves against feelings of overwhelming complexity, demoralization, and helplessness by recourse to idealization or denigration of the physician. Physicians, on the other hand, also need to protect themselves from feelings of grief and helplessness made worse by an overriding sense of their ever-present potential for making a fatal error (Hilfiker, 1985). In this context of heightened emotions and defensive responses, the stereotypic encounter is characterized as a retreat from rational, logical communication on the part of the patient, and a retreat to pure rationalism—to the "science" of medicine—on the part of the physician.

A necessary perspective on this quite dramatic portrait is gained by recognizing that most of the illnesses seen in medical encounters are not the extreme kind. Clinically urgent and very frightening diseases are in fact the exception in everyday practice. Moreover, even these most severe illnesses tend to lead to routine, maintenance-centered encounters over time (Szasz & Hollender, 1956; Tuckett, Boulton, Olson, & Williams, 1985). Despite a reality reflecting a rather undramatic routine, the illusion of drama remains and subverts the talk that explores everyday matters of concern.

The denigration of talk between doctors and patients acts to restrict the many therapeutic purposes it serves. For the patient the talk of the visit gives meaning to feelings of fear and physical discomfort; just naming a medical condition helps enormously in this regard. Through talk, doctors and patients express who they are, what they expect of each other, and what kind of relationship they have. And talk has powerful consequences. A patient's very motivation to get well can be seen as springing from the quality of exchange with the doctor. Physicians need talk as well. Diagnosis can be extremely misguided without adequate talk. Without it, patient and doctor may never even reach a common understanding of the purpose of the medical visit.

Because of deficiencies in talk, the routine medical visit does not nearly reach its therapeutic potential, in which diagnosis can be more accurate, medical intervention more effective, recovery more speedy, realization of quality of life more full, and satisfaction for both doctor and patient more likely. What is wrong is not simply a matter of fault. As we will explore in this book, the patient-physician relationship is burdened on both sides by deep-seated stereotypes and traditions. Although it is debatable whether the relationship ever really served its patients and practitioners as well as nostalgic recollections of the good old days maintain, there is little doubt that it is less than perfectly suited to contemporary needs. The challenge is to understand better and then reshape the relationship so that it may indeed achieve its healing potential.

Our purpose in writing this book is to demonstrate that the talk of the medical visit can be changed for the better and that in itself can transform the way in which medicine is practiced. The positive changes advocated here can be summarized in seven communication-transforming principles: (1) communication should serve the patient's need to tell the story of his or her illness and the doctor's need to hear it; (2) communication should reflect the special expertise and insight that the patient has into his or her physical state and well-being; (3) communication should reflect and respect the relationship between a patient's mental state and his or her physical experience of illness; (4) communication should maximize the usefulness of the physician's expertise; (5) communication should acknowledge and attend to its emotional content; (6) communication should openly reflect the principle of reciprocity, in which the fulfillment of expectations is negotiated; and (7) communication should help participants overcome stereotyped roles and expectations so that both participants gain a sense of power and the freedom to change within the medical encounter.

These communication principles will be described in some detail in the remainder of this chapter and will provide themes that run through the entire book. They are critical for a transformed medical practice and a better model of doctor-patient communication.

THE IMPORTANCE OF TELLING THE STORY

The doctor-patient relationship is different from others. People expect doctors to know them in a fundamental and intimate way, and doctors need to know their patients in order to truly care and cure. This is the first communication principle:

> Communication should serve the patient's need to tell the story of his or her illness and the doctor's need to hear it. Telling of the story is the method by which the meaning of the illness and the meaning of the disease are integrated and interpreted by both doctor and patient.

Patients need to feel that their doctor takes a personal interest in them as individuals, likes them, is concerned and committed to their welfare, and will consequently take pains to do a good job. The fulfillment of the basic need to feel known and understood begins with the telling of the patient's story. Telling one's story can also be therapeutic in its own right in providing a cathartic release and the opportunity for insight and perspective. For physicians, the patient story provides the context for clinical insight necessary for understanding and interpreting the many symptoms and clues the patient provides.

The arithmetic of each physician having an average of 2,500 patients does not equal the experience of each of those 2,500 patients with his or her doctor. Each patient expects that treatment will be uniquely suited to individual needs, but must express these needs within the constraints of short appointment blocks several times throughout the year. It is in this context that patients attempt to establish their unique identity—where patients search for the opportunity to tell their story and to experience the feeling that their story is heard.

But the telling is not so easy. Stories may not be told because patients may fear that they do not meet the standards of life and death intensity they assume their doctors demand. This is unfortunate—especially so because the patient's assumption that the doctor is not interested or that the story is unimportant is infrequently addressed in an explicit manner. If the doctor does not facilitate the story telling—if the patient is not encouraged to go on—he or she very often will not.

The story-telling process is best facilitated when there are no strict limits on patient response. The patient story is not limited to the first and presenting problem. Patients often state a medical complaint as a "ticket of entry" to medical care, even though the primary and most pressing concern may be unrelated to this complaint.

A study focusing on the first ninety seconds of the medical visit found that the patient's response to the physician's opening question was completed in only 23% of the visits studied. In 69% of the visits, the physician interrupted the patient's opening statement after an average of only fifteen seconds to follow up on a stated problem. In only one of these visits was the patient given the opportunity to return to, and complete, the opening statement. For those 30% of patients who were allowed to continue, none of their statements took more than two and a half minutes (Beckman & Frankel, 1984). A later analysis of the concerns raised by patients throughout the visit found that the first-named concern was no more clinically significant than concerns expressed later. However, later concerns tended to be raised in a haphazard manner and received inconsistent attention (Beckman, Frankel, & Darnley, 1985).

Because of embarrassment, fear of appearing foolish, or real anxiety about the possible meaning of symptoms, these other concerns are often hidden beneath the surface of seemingly more legitimate medical complaints. The unstated concerns have been referred to as the patient's hidden agenda, and are especially troublesome for physicians when they surface as the patient is leaving, as an aside (Stoeckle & Barsky, 1981). The dreaded doorway question—"By the way doctor, I have chest tightness (a lump in my breast, swelling in my legs, some problems remembering things, etc.). That's nothing to worry about, right?"—will often necessitate a time-consuming extension of the medical visit.

Another element of story telling is an exploration of the significance and impact of the illness or medical problem for the patient. How patients understand their disease and the attributions they make are extremely important in understanding reactions and fears. Inordinate distress, for example, may stem more from patients' beliefs about what is wrong than from the disease itself. Most patients suspect some specific causative factor for their symptoms or condition. Knowledge of the patient's attribution can be helpful in that it may reveal some of the patient's personal and emotional experience, which may be what is prompting the visit. However, a patient may be reluctant at first to volunteer his or her suspicions for fear of appearing ignorant or foolish. The patient may have an incorrect biomechanical explanation for the symptoms and need education and explanation, or subscribe to religious or cultural beliefs that are at odds with a "scientific explanation." Once these beliefs are out in the open, then some middle ground and accommodation may be reached.

Most patients also have particular expectations in mind when they visit the doctor, although they may be reluctant to make these known directly. Expectations may be for particular treatments (drugs or tests), administrative help, or most commonly, for a better understanding of the etiology, diagnosis, prognosis, or treatment of their condition and how that relates to their prior experience or the experience of others they know.

All of these things—feeling known and understood, having the opportunity for catharsis, insight, and perspective, as well as conveying the life context of the illness, its meaning, interpretation, and the patient's expectations for care—are part of the story the patient tells.

PATIENTS AS EXPERTS

This brings us to a second communication-transforming principle:

The patient should be considered an expert in his or her own right and as such has unique perspectives and valuable insights into his or her physical state, functional status, and quality of life.

In studies of over 23,000 people (Idler & Kasl, 1991) investigators concluded that a simple self-evaluation of health—the answer to the question, "At the present time, how would you rate your health?"—provides strong clues to patient survival over periods as long as seventeen years. Furthermore, people's self-evaluations of health were stronger predictors of death than supposedly objective indicators of health, including detailed physical exams and batteries of tests.

Professional recognition of the importance of patient self-rating of health has only recently emerged. The first studies in this area were done in an attempt to assess "subjective" patient ratings of their own health versus the gold standard of physicians' "objective" ratings. The assumption was that a physician's insight into the health of an individual was more clinically accurate than the individual's own insight. After all, physicians are trained to make health assessments, and have a wide array of sophisticated technology at their disposal. However, since self-evaluations were so frequently asked for in health surveys, there was some interest in determining how valid they were—that is, how close they matched physicians' evaluations.

The predominant findings were that self-ratings and physician ratings of an individual's health were similar in the majority of cases; however, the relationship was far from perfect, with significant differences quite common. Discrepancies in patient and physician ratings were most often the result of patient "health optimism." Patients were two to three times more likely to rate their health better than their physicians rated it. When the opposite was the case, however, and patients' self-ratings of health were poor, researchers found an increased likelihood of impending death. Elderly patients in the Yale Health and Aging Project (Idler & Kasl, 1991) who rated their health as poor were three to six times (females and males, respectively) more likely to die within the four-year follow-up period than those who rated their health as excellent. This risk remained even when a host of objective factors such as the number of health problems, disability, and health risk factors were taken into account. It appears that self-rated health has a unique, predictive, and largely unexplained relationship with death and survival, and that this relationship is more predictive than any prognosis a doctor can provide.

Why would self-evaluations of present health predict future mortality so well, and better than physician assessments? No one really knows. The authors of the Yale Health and Aging Project suggest two explanations. First, it is possible that there is a direct effect of health optimism or pessimism on subsequent health. Individuals who believe themselves to be healthy then act healthy, and indeed become more healthy over time; those who believe themselves to be sick act sick and indeed become sick. The second possibility is that self-evaluations reflect a calculation of life expectancy based on a broad range of information known only to the individual. This might include such objective things as his or her family's chronic disease history, longevity of parents and grandparents, or more subjective feelings—energy and well-being.

Another explanation for these results has focused on judgments of quality of life. Physicians tend to associate general health ratings with the number and severity of chronic conditions, irrespective of the effect of these conditions on the patient's quality of life. However, the impact of disability associated with health conditions is highly variable and contingent not only on individuals themselves, but on their social networks and resources. This includes family, friends, and neighbors who supply help in its many forms, through social contact, direct services, money, and emotional support to enhance an individual's ability to cope with and adapt to physical, social, and environmental challenges. The process of adaptation reflects a daily experience of quality of life. Self-evaluations of health are largely associated with this aspect of living, which is not necessarily known or fully appreciated by physicians—or by family and friends, for that matter.

Indeed, it has been found that patients' and physicians' understandings of overall health differ in basic meaning; physicians rely on medical data while patients draw on physical, functional, social, and emotional aspects of their health (Hall, Epstein, & McNeil, 1989; Martin, Gilson, Bergner, Bobbitt, Pollard, Conn, & Cole, 1976). In the 1989 study, the patients' ratings were related to their functional abilities (such as the ability to walk without a cane or dress oneself), their emotional distress, and the number of different medical diagnoses appearing in their medical charts. It seems the patients appropriately considered overall health to be a broad notion that covered three distinct ways of being healthy. The doctors' ratings, on the other hand, were related mainly to the number of diagnoses the patient had—a much narrower frame of reference. The doctors' understanding of overall health, therefore, seemed constrained by the biomedical point of view (health as defined by medical words in the chart), and not informed by the state of health as the patient experienced it.

Other research on reports of health by patients versus doctors, nurses, or family members also shows disparities between points of view, and the disparities take a curiously similar form. Hospitalized patients report themselves as functioning better than their nurses report; elderly people report themselves as less emotionally distressed than a proxy respondent (usually a family member) reports; and patients have reported themselves to be less depressed than their doctors say they are (Rubenstein, Schairer, Wieland, & Kane, 1984; Yager & Linn, 1981; Epstein, Hall, Tognetti, Son, & Conant, 1989). As in the Idler and Kasl study, patients report feeling healthier than observers would say they are.

These studies reveal gaps in mutual understanding that probably go unrecognized, consciously at least, by everyone but the few researchers who tease them out. Patients typically interact with doctors, nurses, and loved ones with blithe confidence that they are understood, and these others undoubtedly feel they do understand. Where the discrepancies come from is unknown; patients may deny their disabilities, or caregivers may exaggerate them. Possibly, other people think a patient is doing worse than the patient thinks because the patient tends to communicate negative feelings and experiences more often than positive ones. In any case, it is obvious that providers, family, and patients do not share a common understanding of the patient's experience of health and illness.

The famous dictum of the nineteenth-century physician Sir William Osler, "Listen to the patient, he is telling you the diagnosis" (Osler, 1904), is echoed by the conclusions of the Yale researchers: "Knowledge that expressions of subjective health status are sensitive indications of survival length should engender new respect among health professionals for what people, especially the elderly people they treat, are saying about their health" (Idler & Kasl, 1991, p. S65).

BEYOND BIOMEDICINE TO PATIENT EXPERIENCE OF LIFE

The third communication-transforming principle is:

Communication should facilitate recognition of the link between a patient's mental state and the physical experience of illness. Communication should go beyond biomedicine to reflect and respect the patient's experience of life.

Many—in fact, most—medical symptoms for which patients seek medical care cannot be tied to a specific diagnosis. The reason for this failure is that these are not symptoms of disease in the medical sense but are reactions to life. Headaches, rashes, dizziness, fatigue, stomach disorders, aches, chronic constipation or diarrhea, and weight fluctuations may very well portend problems of living rather than underlying disease. People experience stress every day and in every circumstance—certainly everyone has suffered at some time over family relationships, stressful jobs, or money. It is not uncommon for patients to express their distress in genuine physical symptoms such as those listed above. People experiencing life stresses are very high users of health services for physical complaints that are never linked to any organic problem; in fact, these patients take the lion's share of physicians' time.

What is most frustrating for patients experiencing physical symptoms related to life stresses is how difficult it is to communicate these problems to their physician. While patients may be describing their experience from the perspective of their "lifeworld" (Mishler, 1984), physicians are interpreting symptoms from their technological perspective. A patient may feel discouraged from talking about "nonmedical" things such as stress because this may not seem appropriate (or important enough) for the medical encounter, or because of a perception that the doctor can't do anything about it anyway.

Both patients and physicians need to know this is not the case. Through the talk of the medical visit, the doctor and patient can often find effective ways to address the physical manifestation, as well as the contributing underlying distress. Rather than being an irritating distraction from the "business of medicine," problems with emotional and stress dimensions constitute a major component on medical practice. As pointed out by White (1988) in his summary of the literature of medical efficacy, it is exactly these cases, these "distractions," that are the mainstay of medicine. White maintains that about a quarter of all benefits to be derived from medical care cannot be attributed either to technical expertise and agents or to the placebo or Hawthorne effect. White attributes this unnamed mysterious power to the therapeutic power of talk to address and resolve patient problems.

PHYSICIAN AS EXPERT

A singularly consistent finding in studies of doctors and patients conducted over the past twenty-five years has been that patients want as much information as possible from their physicians. And this is the fourth communication-enhancing principle:

Physicians have the duty to share their medical expertise with patients in such a way that this information is clear, relevant, and useful to patients.

The first definition for *doctor* in Webster's is *teacher*. The word teacher implies helping, but this help is not limited to the usual clinical sense of providing correct diagnosis and treatment, or empathy and reassurance. A teacher helps by equipping learners with what they need to help themselves; this includes not just information but also confidence in the value of their own contributions. The educator model is thus more egalitarian and collaborative than the traditional doctor-patient model, and as such is well suited to a literate and consumerist society such as ours.

Paulo Freire (1970), a well-known educator, describes the traditional model of education, in which teachers deposit knowledge and directives for living into passive recipients as though they were empty vessels or bank accounts; he calls this the "banking" method of education. Freire advocates instead a relationship of teacher to learner that acknowledges what learners can impart to teachers. Thus, his model is one in which learning goes both ways and the teacher-learner distinction is considerably blurred.

Applying this to the doctor-patient relationship, one can imagine greater mutual recognition of the unique store of knowledge possessed by the patient, which can be as crucial for a positive treatment outcome as the physician's biomedical knowledge. The medical visit is truly a "meeting between experts" (Tuckett et al., 1985). Even if one prefers the more traditional conception of the doctor alone as the expert, the doctor still has the responsibility to educate patients. Most doctors do recognize this up to a point, but a critical difference between our conception of a true educator and the traditional doctor model is that the educator, by considering the patient's expertise, can share knowledge in a way that is most meaningful to the patient. While we are not suggesting that physicians should try to share the most technical aspects of their knowledge with patients, it is the case that the knowledge most pertinent to most patients' conditions is easily conveyed and readily understood. The imparting of this information creates a spirit of collegiality that enhances patients' ability and willingness to make informed decisions and meaningful commitments to treatment.

A good case in point is the tremendous problem of patient noncompliance—failure to do what the doctor says. Studies of noncompliance report that 10% to 90% of patients do not fully follow doctor's orders; most researchers agree that at least half of all patients do not take their prescribed drugs correctly (Haynes, Taylor, & Sackett, 1981). Adherence to diet, exercise, alcohol restrictions, and other lifestyle changes is probably far worse.

The extent of noncompliance is much more widespread than most doctors estimate, and their appreciation for the problems that lead to noncompliance is very often simplistic. For example, when dealing with patients whose high blood pressure remains uncontrolled, too often the focus is persistently on drugs; the task is to find the right one, the one with proper biochemical composition. But a more fruitful search would be for a better understanding of the patient rather than the drug. Does the patient indeed take the drugs as prescribed? What is the patient's perspective on high blood pressure? Is it viewed as a meaningless measurement associated with nonsymptoms that (illogically) led to a need for drugs? Does the patient see no reason to continue to take the drug when he or she feels well? Does the patient stop if he or she feels worse? Are there side effects that interfere with valued social activities? Are the drugs too expensive?

Attention to these kinds of issues might lead not only to more accurate assessment of the extent of compliance, but also to a negotiation between doctor and patient regarding the most appropriate treatment plan. The result would therefore be not only a concrete plan but a "customer approach to patienthood" that is much more likely to lead to compliance because the treatment plan makes sense to patients and is compatible with their lifestyles (Lazare, Eisenthal, & Wasserman, 1975). Moreover, the result is also likely to enhance patients' satisfaction with physicians. If patients like their physicians and trust not only their technical skill but also their commitment to advocate a plan of treatment that really is best suited for the patients, they are more likely to comply. The physician's negotiating behavior, the full and open exchange of ideas, is the ground from which springs the patient's motivation to comply.

INFORMATION CARRIES EMOTIONAL CONTENT

Though patients certainly want as much information as possible from their physicians, information is not all that patients want. Physicians are not simply expert consultants, although they are that; they are also someone to whom people go when they are particularly vulnerable. People depend on this relationship to be in their best interest, trusting that the doctor is indeed on their side. The fifth communication-transforming principle is:

The exchange of information carries both cognitive and emotional significance.

Patients need factual information as a basis for rational behavior: for example, they can't take drugs intelligently if they don't know about the dosage and side effects. But they also need information for the reduction of uncertainty and anxiety. Further, physicians who provide adequate information are likely to be interpreted as being competent and caring. These interpretations may be a major influence on the doctor-patient relationship and on the entire course of illness, more important even than the information itself.

Most talk during the medical visit consists of giving information or asking questions, with relatively little direct expression of emotions and feelings. This, of course, is not the full picture of the medical exchange, for the nonverbal channels of facial expression, voice quality, posture, touch, gaze, and so forth constantly communicate feelings even when the spoken words may not seem to have any particular emotional content. Feelings get introduced in another way as well. Patients draw conclusions about the doctor— what kind of a person the doctor is, and the nature of the doctor's attitudes and intentions toward the patient—from the totality of doctor behavior. Thus, a doctor who spends all of his or her time on medical business may still inspire good feelings in a patient because the patient values being taken seriously. The patient may infer that the doctor cares a lot because the doctor went to the trouble to be thorough, informative, and accurate.

In fact, all exchanges between doctors and patients carry cues about feelings and attitudes. People emit cues that are given meaning whether they want to or not. Thus, a distressed patient who tries to conceal her agitation may "leak" such cues anyway. A physician who equates professionalism with a neutral demeanor and emotional distance will most likely react in spontaneous expressive ways in spite of these intentions—for example, by revealing irritation with a particularly troublesome patient. And even if a physician is able to be consistently unexpressive, a patient may well interpret that lack of expression not as neutrality but as aloofness, lack of interest, or even as a sign that important information is being withheld. The doctor-patient interaction can be as emotionally laden as any other relationship, and more so than some because of the anxiety that is often brought on by the illness experience and the patient's hypersensitivity to cues given off by the physician.

RECIPROCITY

Negotiation and bargaining are implicit in any relationship, including that of doctor and patient. The sixth communication principle is based on this notion of reciprocity:

> Doctors and patients continually evaluate the adequacy of each other's performance, according to their own values and expectations, and respond in a way that they feel somehow matches with, or is deserved by, the other's behavior.

The common notion of reciprocity centers on things people can do for, or give to, each other in a spirit of exchange. This exchange includes both feelings and calculation. In medical encounters, there seems to be a trade-off between good feelings and coolly calculated obligation. When feelings of gratitude, love, or esteem are strong, a sense of obligation is scarcely felt, and the desire to do something for another feels spontaneous: a deed is done because one wants to. But when positive feelings are not so strong, a sense of obligation emerges, and reciprocity becomes a duty, something one should do. Under these circumstances, awareness of calculation is likely to be high, and calculation of what is due can be exceedingly detailed.

In the medical relationship a special case exists with regard to reciprocity. Doctors can do things for patients, but patients can do things both for doctors and for themselves. Because patients can choose between doctor-directed responses and responses on their own behalf, patients can hurt themselves. As an example, if a physician fails to provide a patient with a preferred drug, the patient may reciprocate disappointment with less than full compliance in taking the drug that was prescribed, or by dropping out of care altogether, even though these actions ultimately hurt only the patient. Reciprocity may work the other way as well. The doctor who is perceived as working especially hard may find that the patient not only expresses gratitude, but also follows the prescribed regimen with special conscientiousness.

Reciprocation can also be literal: payment of bills is expected. But many patients go beyond the expected payment by providing their doctors with gifts, particularly at Christmas, on special occasions, and after a serious illness (Drew, Stoeckle, & Billings, 1983). Patients who feel they did not receive the kind of care they expected may withhold payment of bills, boycott further services, discourage friends from going to this doctor, or even file malpractice suits. The psychological experience of the reciprocity norm in the doctor-patient relationship takes the form of each deciding what form of response or behavior is justified and deserved under the circumstances. Thus minor disappointments might result in partial withholding of payment, but larger disappointments might result in more drastic action.

Although dramatic gestures such as those mentioned above clearly illustrate the reciprocity rule, more subtle reactions as well as moment-to-moment acts within the medical visit can also be seen in this light. Positive statements or facial expressions by the doctor are likely to produce the same behavior in the patient. If a warm greeting pleases the patient, the patient returns good feeling (warm behavior) to the doctor. If one participant behaves in a reserved manner, chances are the other will behave coolly too. Behaviors that are more task-oriented in both doctor and patient can also show reciprocity; for example, more giving of information by the doctor and greater expertise produce better understanding and better patient compliance. Although some of these benefits are fostered directly by the information, we think an equally important force is the motive to repay that is aroused by the patient's perception of good doctor performance. It is also likely that the reciprocation of task-oriented behaviors by other task-oriented behaviors is fostered when a positive emotional climate exists between the doctor and patient.

Reciprocity can also occur when the doctor's and patient's behaviors look quite different on the surface. For example, a patient may respond with liking (an emotional reaction) to a doctor who is highly competent (a technical skill). Such a reaction would be reciprocity if, as mentioned above, the patient interprets such a doctor to be showing his or her own liking or respect for the patient by being so conscientious. What does not happen much is the reverse—a patient making a competence attribution based on the doctor's friendly personal style.

Just this point was made through an experiment by Willson and McNamara (1982), which showed that people viewing taped vignettes of doctor-patient interactions interpreted a competent doctor to be courteous, but did not interpret a courteous one to be competent unless actual competence was portrayed. Courtesy and friendliness were not enough to convince patients of the doctor's expertise, or sufficient to guarantee commitment to the recommended regimen. Patients are constantly making inferences about doctors, and doctors would do well to consider the impact of what they do and say on their patients.

Patients, for their part, need to be persuaded perhaps more than their doctors do that they are important influencers too. The prime fact about social interaction is that people influence each other, and this means that influence in the medical visit is a two-way street. Doctors are profoundly influenced by the demeanor, comments, attitudes, interest, and positive or negative regard expressed by their patients.

That influence can return to help or to haunt the patient. To take an extreme case, a patient who is consistently rude and irritable will almost certainly not receive the same medical care as a patient who conveys more positive or at least constructive attitudes. More subtly, patients' expectations for how their physicians are going to act will very likely come true because the expectation shapes the patient's behavior, which, by reciprocity, is reflected back in the behavior of the doctor. People often invite or even demand a certain manner or attitude in another, without ever knowing they have done so. It is a sad fact that the disappointing or objectionable behavior of others can be so often of our own making.

CONFORMING TO NOTIONS OF "GOOD" DOCTOR AND "GOOD" PATIENT

Just as doctors and patients influence each other, so are they influenced by prior experiences whose impact they bring to the medical visit. The seventh communication-transforming principle is:

Becoming more aware of roles, and the assumptions and expectations they bring with them, can help both participants gain a sense of power and the freedom to change within the medical encounter.

Once learned, both doctor and patient roles are hard to change. One reason lies in the unconscious nature of this kind of social interaction. Like speaking a well-rehearsed part or driving a car, the many words and actions that make up "acting like a doctor" and "acting like a patient" become automatic and escape our awareness.

One reason why people conform to the roles they are cast in is their practically mortal fear of committing social improprieties. This is especially pertinent to the patient role, which traditionally has been a rather passive one. We believe it is often dread of being inappropriate, of doing the wrong thing, that prevents patients from asking more questions or requesting to see their medical charts, even when such actions are clearly in the patients' best interest. Patients feel they are not supposed to do these things.

A different, but nonetheless limiting, attitude patients often have is that the situation itself is a given—a "that's how it is" approach in which patients can do little more than fit in. Attendant on this passivity is the fear that failure to fit in will get one branded as a troublemaker or a crank. Extreme deviance would certainly produce bad effects in any social situation where norms are well established. But patients have more latitude than they think. As they prefer, they can ask more questions, demand more information, take control of certain decisions, read their charts, and in general use fully the time that they are paying for.

Especially for patients, the awareness of roles can help liberate them from feeling they have to act in certain ways. Roles, after all, are just a kind of conformity, not a moral code or rule of law. A good illustration of patient influence involves a man who took his frightened young son to an emergency room with a bad facial cut and announced that he would only see a doctor who was a parent. Such a doctor was found, and the doctor, of course, knew why the demand was made: he could use parenting as well as medical expertise to calm the child and help the father with the tough decision of whether or not to stitch. Interestingly, this kind of assertiveness in the patient's interest probably comes easier when it is on another's behalf, especially a child's. The parent observed that if it were his own face that was bleeding, he probably would have just shrugged and said, "Do what you have to."

While the patient role is learned throughout life, the doctor role is learned in medical school. Medical education is designed not only to teach biochemistry and physiology but to teach how one acts as a doctor. Unfortunately, the current training process is often dehumanizing; interns are forced to give up any semblance of a normal home life and typically work every other night at the hospital (Klass, 1987). This cannot help but create a callous view of patients: they are but one more obstacle to seeing one's family or getting some sleep. Even after training, many doctors feel their lives are unreasonably burdened by the stress of on-call responsibilities and hospital pressures. These experiences can carry over into the medical visit in negative ways (Hilfiker, 1985).

The process of medical education could be changed to provide a more positive experience for young doctors. As we see it, medical education can have two kinds of impact on doctor-patient relations. First, it can affect skills. Medical school can teach doctors to do a variety of things better—to be better communicators and patient educators, to motivate patients more effectively, and to reassure and comfort them better. Second, it can help them think holistically about the kind of doctor they want to be. Critics of medical education have often argued that the emphasis on basic science is out of proportion with its relevance to clinical practice, and that interpersonal and communication skills, which are so critical, get short shrift in the medical curriculum. Indeed, in their early years of medical school, students do a better job of talking with their patients than fully trained doctors do.

A well-known study of medical education found that medical students' interpersonal skills with patients declined as their medical education progressed (Helfer, 1970). This was particularly true for the student's ability to take a good social history. It seems that as students learned more about the science of medicine they found it harder simply to talk with patients, and came to devalue this kind of activity. What were easy exchanges during the first years became an awkward and unproductive series of closed-ended, usually yes-no, questions later on. No doubt related to this narrowing of focus, Martin et al. (1976) found that as training progressed, physicians seemed increasingly to lose their grasp on the patient's total health picture and to focus more and more on biomedical issues.

Although the improvement of physicians' skills in interviewing is valuable, skill does not go to the heart of the matter. Medical school needs to do a better job of inculcating different attitudes in young doctors—in defining for them what is truly important about being a doctor and what are effective, and humane, doctor-patient roles. Our society must figure out how to influence their attitudes so that they come to value certain aspects of patient care differently. Then, of course, when these doctors become mentors themselves, they will provide a different kind of example to their students. If physicians saw themselves more as patient educators, medical education would be different, and the profession would engage in a different kind of self-scrutiny. More attention would be paid to the education of patients, which would translate into more sensitive involvement of doctors in the process of healing.

Taken as a whole these seven principles provide a blueprint for the communication field. They represent the challenges and the potential for a transformation not only in talk but in the clinical model that underlies the practice of medicine.

REFERENCES

Beckman, H. B., & Frankel, R. M. (1984). The effect of physician behavior on the collection of data. *Annals of Internal Medicine, 101*, 692–696.

Beckman, H. B., Frankel, R. M., & Darnley, J. (1985). Soliciting the patient's complete agenda: A relationship to the distribution of concerns. *Clinical Research, 33*, 714A.

Drew, J., Stoeckle, J. D., & Billings, J. A. (1983). Tips, status and sacrifice: Gift giving in the doctor-patient relationship. *Social Science & Medicine, 17*, 399–404.

Epstein, A. M., Hall, J. A., Tognetti, J., Son, L. H., & Conant, L., Jr. (1989). Using proxies to evaluate quality of life: Can they provide valid information about patients' health status and satisfaction with medical care? *Medical Care, 27*, S91–S98.

Freire, P. (1970). *Pedagogy of the oppressed.* New York: Seabury Press.

Hall, J. A., Epstein, A. M., & McNeil, B. J. (1989). Multidimensionality of health status in an elderly population: Construct validity of a measurement battery. *Medical Care, 27*, S168–S177.

Haynes, R. B., Taylor, D. W., & Sackett, D. L. (Eds.) (1981). *Compliance in health care.* 2nd ed. Baltimore: Johns Hopkins University Press.

Helfer, R. E. (1970). An objective comparison of the pediatric interviewing skills of freshman and senior medical students. *Pediatrics, 45*, 623–627.

Hilfiker, D. (1985). *Healing the wounds: A physician looks at his work.* New York: Pantheon.

Idler, E. L., & Kasl, S. V. (1991). Health perceptions and survival: Do global evaluations of health status really predict mortality? *Journal of Gerontology, 46*, S55–S65.

Klass, P. (1987). *A not entirely benign procedure: Four years as a medical student.* New York: Signet.

Lazare, A., Eisenthal, S., & Wasserman, L. (1975). The customer approach to patienthood: Attending to patient requests in a walk-in clinic. *Archives of General Psychiatry, 32*, 553–558.

Martin, D. P., Gilson, B. S., Bergner, M., Bobbitt, R. A., Pollard, W. E., Conn, J. R., & Cole, W. A. (1976). The Sickness Impact Profile: Potential use of a health status instrument for physician training. *Journal of Medical Education, 51*, 942–947.

Mishler, E. G. (1984). *The discourse of medicine: Dialectics of medical interviews.* Norwood, N.J.: Ablex.

Osler, W. (1904). The master-word in medicine. In *Aequanimitas, with other addresses to medical students, nurses, and practitioners of medicine.* Philadelphia: Blakiston.

Rubenstein, L. Z., Schairer, C., Wieland, G. D., & Kane, R. (1984). Systematic biases in functional status assessment of elderly adults: Effects of different data sources. *Journal of Gerontology, 39,* 686–691.

Shorter, E. (1985). *Bedside manners.* New York: Simon and Schuster.

Stoeckle, J. D., & Barsky, A. (1981). Attributions: Uses of social science knowledge in doctoring in primary care. In Eisenberg, L., & Kleinman, A. (Eds.), *The relevance of social science for medicine.* Boston: D. Reidel.

Szasz, P. S., & Hollender, M. H. (1956). A contribution to the philosophy of medicine: The basic model of the doctor-patient relationship. *Archives of Internal Medicine, 97,* 585–592.

Tuckett, D., Boulton, M., Olson, C., & Williams, A. (1985). *Meetings between experts.* New York: Tavistock Publications.

White, K. L. (1988). *The task of medicine: Dialogue at Wickenburg.* Menlo Park, Calif.: Henry J. Kaiser Family Foundation.

Willson, P., & McNamara, J. R. (1982). How perceptions of a simulated physician-patient interaction influence intended satisfaction and compliance. *Social Science & Medicine, 16,* 1699–1703.

Yager, J., & Linn, L. S. (1981). Physician-patient agreement about depression: Notation in medical records. *General Hospital Psychiatry, 3,* 271–276.

2

Models of the Doctor-Patient Relationship

Once the patient and physician are brought together, they enter a relationship predicated on the expectations each holds for the conduct of the other. The relationship thus formed has substantial implications for how the curing and caring process will be accomplished and the extent to which needs and expectations will be met, satisfaction achieved, and health restored.

Critical to expectations regarding the conduct of the medical visit are varying perspectives on notions of authority and autonomy. Medical authority is viewed as part and parcel of the services of an expert—a patient follows the doctor's orders because it is assumed that the orders are scientifically based and well-meaning (Parsons, 1951, 1975). The physician's authority to direct patient behavior is conceded and thus legitimated by patients in light of the physician's advanced training and expertise. On occasion, however, patients may resist doctor's orders and declare an intention to follow their own inclinations instead. This withdrawal of authority can be seen as an expression of patient autonomy—the power to resist the physician's will (Haug & Lavin, 1983).

There are two views regarding the potential clash between patient autonomy and physician authority in the doctor-patient relationship. The first is a consensual accommodation and the second is outright conflict. The consensual view has been articulated by Talcott Parsons (1951, 1975), who argues that conflict is managed and diffused by well-defined societal expectations for both patient and physician conduct.

In contrast, Freidson (1970b) sees conflict as ongoing and fundamental to the doctor-patient relationship. The most fully discussed area of conflict related to the autonomy/authority clash is in regard to medical knowledge. In some respects the argument over knowledge may be reduced to a question of ownership.

Parsons argues that inherent in the definition of a physician is the dedication of a lifetime to mastery of knowledge and the gaining of experience in the application of that knowledge. The fund of medical knowledge is so vast and complex, the schooling so intense and grueling, and the daily experience so unique, that an unbridgeable competence gap exists between physicians and the lay world. Medical knowledge is thus earned and owned by doctors. Moreover, this knowledge is impossible to share. There are protections afforded patients since they must accept medical practice on faith. Central to this protection is a higher order of moral conduct that physicians are held to, including a code of ethics defining the special duty of physicians to protect the interests of their patients.

Patients, for their part, rely on physician adherence to this moral code and therefore cooperate with doctor's orders. Any conflict between doctor and patient is resolved by physician authority and the assumption that "the doctor knows best." A patient who resists doctor's orders risks potential loss of standing as a patient and being labeled a malingerer or a fake; no patient can truly want to get well if he or she does not cooperate with the doctor.

A different view regarding medical knowledge, physician authority, and patient autonomy is articulated by Freidson (1960). While agreeing with Parsons that the predominant characteristic of the physician is the mastery of expert knowledge and experience, Freidson sees the disinclination of physicians to share information with patients less as a function of a competence gap than as a safeguard for high status and professional standing. Moreover, a less knowledgeable patient is less likely to second-guess the doctor or detect medical errors (Freidson, 1970b).

In any given situation, a patient may fear that the physician has overlooked or denigrated a significant and important symptom because the physician's knowledge is flawed or incomplete. This may either be because of deficiencies in medical science or because of the personal failings of the physician (Freidson, 1960). The calculus of only one physician relating to many patients raises the specter that the physician cannot always give sufficient attention or time to every patient or medical problem. Even if the physician fails only once in ten thousand cases, that is sufficient cause for an individual patient to wonder if his or hers will be that case (Freidson, 1960). A share in the information base can help assure a patient that this is not the case. Moreover, most patients highly value information as a way of coping with the uncertainty of illness and as a mechanism for greater participation in medical decision making. (The value and importance of information to patients are discussed further in Chapter 6.)

Professional knowledge, per se, is not all that is gained during training. Physicians also learn and internalize a worldview that includes a way of thinking based on the biomedical model of disease (Engel, 1977). The predominant view a physician brings to medical practice is one anchored in the world of biochemistry and technology. In contrast, a patient's world is a complex web of personality, culture, living situations, and relationships, all of which color and define the illness experience (Kleinman, 1987; Mishler, 1984). The conflict is between incomplete perspectives: the biomedical view loses the context of the patient's life, while the patient's experience may lack insight into science and potential medical intervention.

A contest of definitions ensues between doctor and patient. The physician wants a biomedical definition, in terms of a disease with known physical manifestations, which implies medical ownership, while the patient wants the definition to be his or her own in terms of the illness experience (Mishler, 1984; Cassell, 1976). The physician who dismisses a debilitating flu as "only the flu" may miss, from the patient's perspective, the full impact of the illness experience and its meaning. For the patient, the flu may be seen as an indication of a compromised immune system and an early sign of cancer. Failure to appreciate this kind of significance arises from a fundamental difference between doctors and patients in their worldview.

It is through the manipulation of information and the definition of the problem that the nature and conduct of the visit are determined—what will be said and done, when, and how. Patients have some measure of power as to how the medical visit will proceed, although its expression is usually more subtle than that of the physician. Patients can withhold information from the physician—give an untruthful or incomplete report of their medical condition, for instance—to create an impression of being more or less sick than they actually are (Roth, 1963). They can, of course, request and insist on certain procedures or prescriptions, ask questions and probe the physician's clinical reasoning, or refuse to go along with a recommended test or treatment. Direct confrontation between doctor and patient, however, is the exception rather than the rule. Far more common are maneuvers and negotiations that span a broad spectrum of power relations.

It is along this negotiated spectrum that patient autonomy and physician authority are defined in any given relationship. Because of the great variability in patients' ability to negotiate in this realm, ethicists have identified the potential for medical coercion as a central question of medical ethics. Indeed, since the 1960s patient autonomy has become a tenet of medical ethics, and is almost universally regarded as a necessary and important element of civilized and enlightened medical care (President's Commission for the Study of Ethical Problems in Medicine and Biomedical and Behavioral Research, 1982).

Table 2.1
Types of Doctor-Patient Relationships

	Physician Control	
Patient Control	Low	High
Low	Default	Paternalism
High	Consumerism	Mutuality

To explore further the varying perspectives on the doctor-patient relationship, four models of the care relationship will be discussed.

PROTOTYPES OF CONTROL IN THE DOCTOR-PATIENT RELATIONSHIP

The expression of control, and the dynamics of negotiation in the doctor-patient relationship, can take several forms—each shaping a markedly different relationship. Table 2.1 illustrates the four archetypal forms of control in the doctor-patient relationship: paternalism, consumerism, mutuality, and default.

The prototype of paternalism is shown in the upper right quadrant, illustrating a relationship of high physician control and low patient control. In this model of relations, physicians dominate decision making in regard to both information and services; the implication is that these decisions are in the patient's best interest. The patient's job is to cooperate with medical advice, that is, to do what he or she is told.

The lower left quadrant of the table represents consumerism, the opposite extreme to paternalism; here the power relationship between doctors and patients is reversed. Patient demands for information and technical services are accommodated by a cooperating physician. This type of relationship redefines the medical encounter as a marketplace transaction. Caveat emptor, "let the buyer beware," rules the transaction, with power resting in the buyer (patient) who can make the decision to buy (seek care) or not, as he or she sees fit (Haug & Lavin, 1983).

While still stressing patient control, the prototype of mutuality shown in the lower right quadrant proposes a more moderate alternative to the polar extremes of paternalism and consumerism. In mutuality, each participant brings strengths and resources to the relationship on a relatively even footing. Inasmuch as power in the relationship is balanced, decisions are the result of what may be considered a meeting between equals. The patient's job, in this model, is to become part of a joint venture.

What happens when patient and physician expectations are at odds or when the need for change in the relationship cannot be negotiated? A possible consequence of poor fit, or the failure to change the relationship as needs and circumstances change, is relationship default, represented in the upper left of the table and characterized by a total lack of control. It is in this case that a patient may drop out of care completely because of failed expectations or frustrated goals.

Contrasting perspectives from the research literature have been drawn to illustrate each of the four prototypes.

PATERNALISM

Paternalism is widely regarded as the traditional form of the doctor-patient relationship, and it is still seen as the most common one (Parsons, 1951; Szasz & Hollender, 1956; President's Commission, 1982). A passive patient and dominant physician as the idealized therapeutic relationship is most clearly articulated by Parsons in his classic writings on the sick role (Parsons, 1951). Parsons sees the doctor and patient as fulfilling necessary functions in a well-balanced and well-maintained social structure. Sickness in this model is considered a necessary, occasional respite providing a brief exemption for patients from societal responsibilities. However, for society to continue to function, this respite must be controlled. By defining the terms of the illness and its privileges, physicians provide this controlling force.

When sick, the patient is allowed the privileges of convalescence—the patient is not held responsible for his or her poor health and is excused from everyday responsibilities. However, in order to enjoy these privileges, the patient must seek technically competent help and comply with medical advice. The patient's role is passive and dependent. In contrast, the doctor's role is defined as professionally dominant and autonomous. The doctor legitimates the patient's illness and determines the course of treatment. In doing so, the physician is compelled by professional ethics to act only in his or her sphere of expertise, to maintain an emotional detachment and distance from the patient, and to act in the patient's best interest.

This model is argued to be more functional than others from a societal perspective. The authority afforded physicians provides the weight necessary for the important certification role of physicians in determining how sick a patient is and how much leeway will be given to the patient. This might include exemptions from work and home responsibilities, as well as economic compensation for disabilities associated with work-related accidents. Moreover, it is physicians' authority that gives them their ability to reintegrate patients into society at the end of their sickness episode. The physician is the one who determines when health is restored and sick privileges are withdrawn.

In addition to the social control function that the paternalism model affords, there are significant nurturing and supportive aspects to this type of relationship. Patients may draw comfort and support from a doctor-parent figure. Indeed, the supportive nature of paternalism appears to be all the more important when patients are very sick and at their most vulnerable (Ende, Kazis, Ash, & Moskowitz, 1989; Ende, Kazis, & Moskowitz, 1990). Relief of the burden of worry is curative in itself, some argue, and the trust and confidence implied by this model allow the doctor to perform "medical magic." There is also evidence that idealization of the physician can have an important therapeutic effect, as placebo studies have demonstrated (Lasagna, Mosteller, von Feisinger, & Beecher, 1954).

Relatively little is known about what kinds of patients are likely to prefer more paternalistic relationships with their physicians. Several sociodemographic variables do appear to be associated with relationship preference. The strongest of these is older age, but lower income and lower level of occupation are also associated with this preference (Ende et al., 1989; Haug & Lavin, 1983; Pendleton & House, 1984). Other investigators have suggested that it is the wide gap in educational background and socioeconomic status between most patients and physicians that contributes to the deference of lower social class patients and their adoption of a passive and dependent role in the doctor-patient relationship (Waitzkin, 1985; Pratt, Seligmann, & Reader, 1957). Also citing the disparity in status and education between patients and physicians, the President's Commission for the Study of Ethical Problems (1982) concluded that even when patients and physicians have mutually agreed upon a paternalistic relationship, questions regarding its appropriateness may still be raised. The commission argued that patients and doctors are often on so unequal a footing that few patients can really play an equal role with physicians in shaping the relationship. The possibility exists, then, that patients may adopt a passive patient role, not fully aware of alternatives or able to negotiate a more active stance.

A difficulty in much of the literature, and in the work cited above, is the wide range regarding how the passive patient role is defined. Several investigators (Ende et al., 1989, 1990; Strull, Lo, & Charles, 1984; Vertinsky, Thompson, & Uyeno, 1974) define the active patient role as including the decision-making prerogative in the therapeutic relationship, and by extension, a passive patient role as patient deference to physicians in decision making. A now well-replicated finding, using this definition, is that patients show rather weak interest in assuming the responsibility for medical decision making (Ende et al., 1989, 1990; Strull et al., 1984; Vertinsky et al., 1974; Pendleton & House, 1984).

While decision-making preference has shown some, though weak, association with sociodemographic and knowledge variables, far stronger relationships have been found with illness severity (Ende et al., 1989, 1990). This suggests that it is being ill that determines decision-making preference, rather than knowledge and social status, as argued earlier. If illness severity is the critical variable, Ende and colleagues hypothesize, then physicians themselves, when under the care of a doctor, would relinquish their autonomy in the same way as other patients.

In studying such a situation, Ende and colleagues (1989, 1990) surveyed 151 physicians and 315 patients attending a university medical clinic on their decision-making preferences. There was a significant but small difference in decision-making preference between the physicians and patients, with physicians having a slightly higher preference for decision making than others (41 versus 34 on a 100-point scale), but their preference was still short of favoring equal participation.

Findings from the study suggest that physicians, like the regular patients in the study, preferred that the principal role in decision making for their illnesses be taken by the doctor, not by themselves (Ende et al., 1990). Moreover, as the severity of illness increased, the tendency of physician-patients was to rely even more on their own physicians for decision making. Because the physicians in this study responded so similarly to patients, the investigators concluded that medical knowledge and sociocultural factors are only minor determinants of patient attitudes toward autonomy, while illness severity appears to play a more critical role.

CONSUMERISM

The advent of medical consumerism in this country has been attributed to several significant societal changes since the 1960s (Reeder, 1972). The first of these is the shift from curative to preventive services. Reeder notes that in a system dominated by curative or emergency care, there is a "seller's market," and the relationship tends to be characterized by the patient's role as supplicant. However, when prevention of illness is emphasized, the patient is less a supplicant than a skeptic. Part of the doctor's job is to convince the patient of the necessity of noncurative services such as periodic check-ups. Under these circumstances, there are elements of a "buyer's market," and a tendency for the "customer to be right."

Another feature of societal change, described by Reeder, is the development of consumerism as a social movement and the redefinition of a person as a consumer rather than a patient. In a similar vein, a concurrent critical focus on the bureaucratization of the system of medical care delivery and its spiraling costs has resulted in increasing use of the term *health care provider* to replace the more traditional *doctor*. Redefinition of the doctor-patient relationship as a consumer-provider exchange is more than a matter of simple semantics, for it refocuses the traditional perspective and thereby changes the very nature of the social relationship between the medical profession and the lay world (Reeder, 1972).

Several authors have defined consumerism as a patient challenge to unilateral decision making by physicians in reaching closure on diagnosis and working out treatment plans (Haug & Lavin, 1983). Inherent in this definition is a challenge to physician authority by reversing the very basic nature of the power relationship: "It focuses on the purchaser's (patient's) rights and seller's (physician's) obligations, rather than on physician's rights (to direct) and patient obligations (to follow directions). . . . In a consumer relationship, the seller has no particular authority; if anything, legitimated power rests in the buyer, who can make the decision to buy or not to buy, as he or she sees fit" (Haug & Lavin, 1981, p. 213).

Because of the marketplace emphasis of consumerism, and societal concern with medical cost, it is not surprising that some investigators have focused consumerist behavior on cost-related issues. An emphasis on the economic ramifications of consumerism has stressed the consumer's role in making cost-conscious choices among insurance options and providers, using services more sparingly, and being more selective in the acceptance of provider advice based on its cost (Hibbard & Weeks, 1987).

An illustrative study of the consumer as cost-conscious health shopper was conducted by Hibbard and Weeks (1985). These investigators interviewed almost 2,000 consumers (half were working-age government employees, and half Medicare enrollees who were over sixty-five years of age) to determine the extent to which they behaved in a consumerist manner. Indications of consumerism were: (a) cost-consciousness—using physician fees as a factor in selecting a physician, choosing not to see a physician when ill because of cost, or asking about fees in discussions with a physician; (b) information-seeking—reading health columns or articles, using health or medical reference books; (c) exercising independent judgment—following doctors' instructions precisely or using one's own judgment in following doctors' orders; and (d) consumer knowledge—response to a six-question consumer sophistication scale.

The investigators report that a minority of respondents engaged in consumer-like behaviors, with 39% of the respondents being classified as cost-sensitive, 37% as health information seekers, and 34% as using independent judgment in following doctors' advice. Moreover, the Medicare population scored substantially lower on all of these indicators than did the working-age population. Overall, the results indicate that those with greater education, as well as those in younger age groups, were most likely to engage in consumerist behaviors. Respondents who reported greater faith in doctors, and more dependence on them, were much less likely than others to adopt a consumerist orientation.

Older respondents appeared especially unwilling to act independent of medical authority and exercise independent judgment. The authors suggest that the older cohorts may have a different perception of the expected and proper patient role in health care. An exception to the elderly deference to physicians, however, was evident among those who had greater experience with the health care system and for whom economic issues held greater salience. Out-of-pocket costs and the perception of health care costs as a burden were associated with all four consumer attributes—even among older, Medicare respondents. In a somewhat similar vein, an earlier study by these investigators found that individuals over the age of fifty-five, particularly females who were well educated and generally skeptical of the medical profession, were more likely to obtain a physician fee guide than other people (Hibbard & Weeks, 1985).

The finding that faith in, and dependency on, physicians was an important barrier to the adoption of a consumerist orientation led the authors to conclude that patients need help not just in learning about cost issues but in making the transition from being the traditional passive patient to being a consumer. This would include stressing less common components of consumerism, such as when to seek care, how to negotiate successfully in the medical encounter, whether or not to accept medical advice, and where to seek alternative sources of information (Hibbard & Weeks, 1987).

An exploration of the extent to which patients are actually adopting a consumerist approach in medical visits, and the nature of physicians' response to such a challenge, was undertaken by Haug and Lavin (1983). Based on a survey of 466 laypeople and 86 physicians, the investigators found that substantial percentages of both the public and physicians (60% and 81%, respectively) espoused attitudes consistent with a consumerist perspective. However, the extent of commitment to a consumerist model dropped when actual behavior was assessed. About half the public reported actual instances of challenging behavior: 30% reported a single instance of confrontation and 17% reported two or more.

Survey respondents who were more rejecting of authority in general, more skeptical of physicians' service orientation, younger, and better educated were more likely to express consumerist attitudes. Reports of consumerist behaviors, however, were more likely to come from those who questioned physician competence, believed medical error occurred in their care, and were younger.

The view from physicians was different. Despite the high level of endorsement for consumerist attitudes, only 8% of physicians indicated that they have accommodated patients' demands for decision-making power. Approximately half the physicians indicated that they used persuasion when challenged to convince a patient of the appropriateness of their recommendation rather than, as the other half, relying on traditional authority. The physicians who were more likely to accommodate patient requests expressed more modern attitudes, including the denigration of authority in general and a belief in the fallibility of the physician. As one might expect, these physicians also held positive views of patients who raise questions.

When things seem to go wrong, when satisfaction is low, or when a patient suspects less than optimal care or outcome, patients are more likely to question physician authority (Ende et al., 1989; Haug & Lavin, 1983; Vertinsky et al., 1974) and to adopt a more active role in the doctor-patient relationship. As is evident from the work described earlier, patients' requests may be negotiated and accommodated or may be perceived as confrontational and critical.

When medical or service requests by the patient are within the boundaries of good medical judgment, and for most conditions these boundaries are set quite wide, accommodation can occur with little conflict. When these demands are contrary to standard practice, however, the physician is skirting the mainstream of medicine and risking ostracism and ridicule by medical colleagues. The reluctance to share decision-making responsibility with patients may be established early, during a physician's training, when heavy stress is put on physician control in order to carry out their medical responsibilities, even over patient objections (Haug & Lavin, 1983).

An example of physician accommodation to patient requests is provided by Norman Cousins's account of his recovery from a rare, life-threatening disease. Cousins relates how, while hospitalized, he presented his physician with his decision to try extremely high doses of vitamin C to treat his disease. He also decided to stop all other medication. Cousins's statement about his doctor is telling:

I was incredibly fortunate to have as my doctor a man who knew that his biggest job was to encourage to the fullest the patient's will to live and to mobilize all the natural resources of body and mind to combat disease. Dr. Hitzig was willing to set aside the large and often hazardous armamentarium of powerful drugs . . . when he became convinced that his patient might have something better to offer. (Cousins, 1979, p. 44)

According to Cousins, his doctor agreed to the course of treatment because he really could offer no alternatives and because he knew that he could best serve his patient by encouraging the will to live and the need to feel some control over his terrible and overwhelming illness.

While this case of physician accommodation seems dramatic, in fact there is little evidence that the more traditional course of treatment in this instance, the likely physician decision, would have been more effective. As noted by Brody (1980), medicine is not an accomplished science. There are tremendous gaps in knowledge. Indeed, it has been estimated that the effectiveness of treatment is unknown for about 90% of medical conditions seen in routine practice (Pickering, 1979). Moreover, many medical decisions are as related to the physician's personality and social characteristics as they are to the nature of the medical problem itself (Eisenberg, 1979).

Besides the substantive aspect of a medical decision, there are also psychological concerns to consider when a physician does not accommodate a patient request. Loss of decision-making control may exacerbate the feelings of helplessness and dependency that often accompany illness, and consequently worsen the patient's clinical prognosis. In their study of patient perception of involvement in decision making, Brody and colleagues (Brody, Miller, Lerman, Smith, & Caputo, 1989) found that patients who reported playing an active role in their medical visit were more satisfied with their physicians, had lower levels of illness concerns, and had a greater sense of control over their illnesses than passive patients. One week after the visit, active patients reported less discomfort, fewer symptoms, and a better overall medical condition than passive patients.

These results are also consistent with a series of studies by Greenfield and associates in which verbally active participation in the medical visit was associated with positive physiological changes in blood sugar control and high blood pressure, as well as improvements in functional status and quality of life measures (Greenfield, Kaplan, & Ware, 1985; Greenfield, Kaplan, Ware, Yano, & Frank, 1988). In a similar vein, Cassileth and associates (Cassileth, Zupkis, Sutton-Smith, & March, 1980) reported that patients who wanted to be involved in treatment decisions were significantly more hopeful than others.

MUTUALITY

In that the physician brings expertise and experience to the medical encounter, but the patient lives with the results, a sharing of decision-making responsibility is reasonable (Herman, 1985). The prototype of mutuality as a model of doctor-patient relations presents a more moderate alternative to the extremes of paternalism and consumerism. The model views the patient neither as standing alone, nor as standing aside, when the difficult task of medical decision making is undertaken. Each of the participants brings strengths and resources to the relationship, as well as a commitment to work through disagreements in a mutually respectful manner.

An illustration of how mutuality may be instituted in the medical encounter is provided by Quill (1983) in detailing his use of a contractual approach to patient care. Inherent in this approach are four underlying assumptions: (1) each participant has unique responsibilities; (2) the relationship is consensual, not obligatory; (3) there is a willingness to negotiate; and (4) each participant must benefit from the relationship. The starting point of the contract is the delineation of the patient's problem(s) and requested intervention. This is a two-way process; the patient needs to define his or her problem in an open and full manner, and the physician needs to work with him or her to articulate the problem and refine the request.

Once expectations are verbalized, a process of negotiation can begin. Some requests can be filled with little difficulty; some requests need only minor modification; some requests require a good deal of compromise, discussion, and debate; and finally, some requests must be denied because they are patently harmful or violate the physician's sense of ethics and good judgment. The patient is free to seek care elsewhere when demands are not satisfactorily met. Likewise, the physician is free to withdraw services formally from a patient if he or she feels it is impossible to satisfy patient demands or achieve treatment objectives.

Brody (1980) has identified four steps by which the physician can encourage mutuality. These are: (1) the establishment of an atmosphere conducive to participation by enhancing the patient's perception that his or her contributions are appropriate and appreciated; (2) the ascertainment of the patient's goals and expectations; (3) the education of the patient about the nature of his or her problem, discussing the pros and cons of alternative evaluation and treatment approaches, and the presentation and explanation of the physician's recommendations; and, finally, (4) the elicitation of the patient's informed suggestions and preferences and the negotiation of any disagreements between physician and patient.

Several authors have suggested that a formal process in which physicians assist patients in stating their values regarding particular decisions is the most desirable method by which a mutual, collaborative exchange may take place (Speedling & Rose, 1985). Deciding on a course of treatment for breast cancer, for example, which might include a radical mastectomy as opposed to a more limited surgery augmented by radiation and chemotherapy, is a decision that can best be made by explicitly working through its implications for a woman's self-image, tolerance of chemotherapy side effects, and issues of sexuality.

On a less formal level this same goal may be achieved through a general process of values clarification directed by the provider. For instance, exploration of values related to health, sexuality, independence, and economics (among others) may have tremendous implications for health practices. Linking methods of treatment to these values may help elucidate dimensions of decision-making and therapeutic commitment for the patient in ways that may be new and constructive.

Engagement in this process may be seen as fulfilling the provider's responsibility in assuring that medical expertise is fully utilized. The prospect of making an important therapeutic decision without guidance and support can be overwhelming to a patient. Decision making cannot be expected to take place within a therapeutic vacuum; real communication is not simply the communication of a treatment catalogue. Meaningful exchange is the give and take necessary for an understanding of the patient's perspective by the provider and an appreciation of the options and their consequences, in terms of daily life, by the patient.

DEFAULT

Relationship default is characterized by a total lack of control by either patient or physician. This circumstance reflects a stagnant situation in which an action-paralysis has occurred. Neither the doctor nor the patient has taken responsibility for medical decisions, and they have not negotiated a mutually acceptable middle ground. This may happen when expectations are at odds or when needs and circumstances have changed so that a once functional relationship is no longer optimal.

A poorly functioning relationship may continue for a long time, without direction, or may terminate without any resolution. It is in this case that a patient may drop out of care completely because of failed expectations or frustrated goals, reflecting bitterly on the unresponsiveness of doctors. Most often the physician will be unaware of the reasons for loss of this patient. Indeed, the physician may not even realize that this patient has dropped out of care, as the patient will simply not come back.

In the worst of scenarios, when a medical outcome has gone bad, the physician may become aware of a failed relationship through a malpractice complaint. While communication difficulties are not often identified as the precipitating cause in malpractice suits, they are widely believed to be the major predisposing cause. Experts on malpractice have concluded that what happens in the office, and the kinds of relationships that are developed there, are critical in setting the stage for a patient's subsequent reaction if there are problems in treatment (Robertson, 1985). It is believed that the majority of malpractice claims would not be pursued if the patient, or the patient's family, were not angered over failures or disappointments in their relationship with the physician (American Medical Association, Special Task Force on Professional Liability and Insurance, 1984–85). In a similar vein, according to a recent survey, nearly two-thirds of physicians who have been sued for malpractice and their patient-litigants thought malpractice could be significantly reduced by improved communication (Shapiro, Simpson, & Lawrence, 1989).

THE DYNAMIC NATURE OF DOCTOR-PATIENT RELATIONSHIPS

Expectations regarding medical authority and patient autonomy are complex; they are often unstated and they are dynamic. The patient's social world, physical condition, stage and type of illness, and a host of cultural and demographic factors have relevance for the kind of relationship a patient desires. As these conditions change, the kind of relationship that works best for a patient may change (Szasz & Hollender, 1956).

In light of the wide variation in patient preferences, it is critical for providers to gain a sense of the level of decision making their individual patients prefer. Moreover, since this may change over time, inquiry should be an ongoing process. The suggestions by Brody (1980) and Quill (1983) mentioned earlier are important ways in which this communication process may be facilitated.

It is easy to suggest that doctors and patients should choose one another by "relationship fit"—a consumerist patient will be happiest with an egalitarian and accommodating physician; a patient who prefers to defer to the physician is best served by a "take-charge" doctor, and so on. However, there are structural and situational constraints that limit the freedom of patients to change doctors at will, or for physicians to dismiss easily their responsibility to patients (Haug & Lavin, 1981). Because of economic constraints or the nature of an unusual medical condition, the doctor and patient may be more deeply committed to one another, and for far longer, than either would like.

But, perhaps a more compelling argument for negotiation and accommodation rather than discontinuity is the likelihood that needs and circumstances will change over time, and that the relationship could better serve both its parties if it had the flexibility to change as well.

REFERENCES

American Medical Association, Special Task Force on Professional Liability and Insurance. (1984–85). Professional liability in the 1980s.

Brody, D. S. (1980). The patient's role in clinical decision making. *Annals of Internal Medicine, 93*, 718–722.

Brody, D. S., Miller, S. M., Lerman, C. E., Smith, D. G., & Caputo, G. C. (1989). Patient perception of involvement in medical care: Relationship to illness attitudes and outcomes. *Journal of General Internal Medicine, 4*, 506–511.

Cassell, E. J. (1976). *The healer's art.* Cambridge, Mass.: MIT Press.

Cassileth, B. R., Zupkis, R. V., Sutton-Smith, K., & March, V. (1980). Information and participation preferences among cancer patients. *Annals of Internal Medicine, 92*, 832–836.

Cousins, N. (1979). *Anatomy of an illness as perceived by the patient.* New York: Norton.

Eisenberg, J. M. (1979). Sociologic influences on decision making by clinicians. *Annals of Internal Medicine, 90*, 957–964.

Ende, J., Kazis, L., Ash, A., & Moskowitz, M. A. (1989). Measuring patients' desire for autonomy: Decision making and information-seeking preferences among medical patients. *Journal of General Internal Medicine, 4*, 23–30.

Ende, J., Kazis, L., & Moskowitz, M. A. (1990). Preferences for autonomy when patients are physicians. *Journal of General Internal Medicine, 5*, 506–509.

Engel, G. L. (1977). The need for a new medical model: A challenge for biomedicine. *Science, 196*, 129–136.

Freidson, E. (1960). Client control and medical practice. *American Journal of Sociology, 65*, 374–382.

Freidson, E. (1970b). *Professional dominance.* Chicago: Aldine Press.

Greenfield, S., Kaplan, S., & Ware, J. E., Jr. (1985). Expanding patient involvement in care: Effects on patient outcomes. *Annals of Internal Medicine, 102*, 520–528.

Greenfield, S., Kaplan, S. H., Ware, J. E., Jr., Yano, E. M., & Frank, H. J. L. (1988). Patients' participation in medical care: Effects on blood sugar control and quality of life in diabetes. *Journal of General Internal Medicine, 3*, 448–457.

Haug, M. R., & Lavin, B. (1981). Practitioner or patient—Who's in charge? *Journal of Health and Social Behavior, 22*, 212–229.

Haug, M., & Lavin, B. (1983). *Consumerism in medicine: Challenging physician authority.* Beverly Hills, Calif.: Sage Publications.

Herman, J. M. (1985). The use of patients' preferences in family practice. *Journal of Family Practice, 20*, 153–156.

Hibbard, J. H., & Weeks, E. C. (1985). Consumer use of physician fee information. *Journal of Health and Human Resources Administration, 7*, 321–335.

Hibbard, J. H., & Weeks, E. C. (1987). Consumerism in health care: Prevalence and predictors. *Medical Care, 25*, 1019–1032.

Kleinman, A. (1987). Explanatory models in health care relationships: A conceptual frame for research on family-based health-care activities in relation to folk and professional forms of clinical care. In Stoeckle, J. (Ed.), *Encounters between patients and doctors*. Cambridge, Mass.: MIT Press.

Lasagna, L., Mosteller, F., von Feisinger, J. M., & Beecher, H. K. (1954). A study of the placebo response. *American Journal of Medicine, 37*, 770–779.

Mishler, E. G. (1984). *The discourse of medicine: Dialectics of medical interviews*. Norwood, N.J.: Ablex.

Parsons, T. (1951). *The social system*. Glencoe, Ill.: The Free Press.

Parsons, T. (1975). The sick role and the role of the physician reconsidered. *Milbank Memorial Fund Quarterly, 53*, 257–278.

Pendleton, L., & House, W. C. (1984). Preferences for treatment approaches in medical care: College students versus diabetic outpatients. *Medical Care, 22*, 644–646.

Pickering, G. (1979). Therapeutics: Art or science? *Journal of the American Medical Association, 242*, 649–653.

Pratt, L., Seligmann, A., & Reader, G. (1957). Physicians' views on the level of medical information among patients. *American Journal of Public Health, 47*, 1277–1283.

President's Commission for the Study of Ethical Problems in Medicine and Biomedical and Behavioral Research. (1982). *Making health care decisions: The ethical and legal implications of informed consent in the patient-practitioner relationship*. Vol. 1. Washington, D.C.: Government Printing Office.

Quill, T. E. (1983). Partnerships in patient care: A contractual approach. *Annals of Internal Medicine, 98*, 228–234.

Reeder, L. G. (1972). The patient-client as a consumer: Some observations on the changing professional-client relationship. *Journal of Health and Social Behavior, 13*, 406–412.

Robertson, W. O. (1985). *Medical malpractice: A preventive approach*. Seattle: University of Washington Press.

Roth, J. A. (1963). Information and the control of treatment in tuberculosis hospitals. In Freidson, E., *The hospital in modern society*. London: Free Press of Glencoe.

Shapiro, R. S., Simpson, D. E., & Lawrence, S. L. (1989). A survey of sued and nonsued physicians and suing patients. *Archives of Internal Medicine, 149*, 2190–2196.

Speedling, E. J., & Rose, D. N. (1985). Building an effective doctor-patient relationship: From patient satisfaction to patient participation. *Social Science & Medicine, 21*, 115–120.

Strull, W. M., Lo, B., & Charles, G. (1984). Do patients want to participate in medical decision making? *Journal of the American Medical Association*, *252*, 2990–2994.

Szasz, P. S., & Hollender, M. H. (1956). A contribution to the philosophy of medicine: The basic model of the doctor-patient relationship. *Archives of Internal Medicine*, *97*, 585–592.

Vertinsky, I. B., Thompson, W. A., & Uyeno, D. (1974). Measuring consumer desire for participation in clinical decision making. *Health Services Research*, *9*, 121–134.

Waitzkin, H. (1985). Information-giving in medical care. *Journal of Health and Social Behavior*, *26*, 81–101.

3

The Influence of Patient Characteristics on Communication between the Doctor and the Patient

It has been argued that the basis of trust between patients and their physicians lies in the physician's dedication to "universalism," that is, the responsibility to treat all patients alike without regard to particular attributes or ascribed traits (Parsons, 1951). It is reasoned that patient care must be universalistic or suspicion and caution would prevail over trust and confidence in the doctor-patient relationship. Fear that physicians might act upon age, class, or racial stereotypes could undermine the fabric of the social contract upon which the therapeutic relation rests. In light of the significance of potential violations of physician universalism, investigation of the association between patient attributes and aspects of care should be a research priority. This is not the case. There have been relatively few methodologically sound studies designed specifically to investigate the role of sociological factors in medical visits (Greene, Adelman, Charon, & Hoffman, 1986; Gerbert, 1984; Roter, Hall, & Katz, 1988).

There are three mechanisms by which one might hypothesize physician behavior to relate to patient characteristics. First, there may be an unintended association between the care process and patient attributes that is produced by mutual ignorance of social or cultural norms. The marked differences that often exist between physicians and their patients (for example, patients who are poor, uneducated, and minorities) may lead to very basic communication difficulties. Citing sociolinguistic theorists, Waitzkin (1985) has generalized to the medical context the finding that middle-class subjects tend to be verbally explicit while working-class subjects tend to communicate more implicitly through nonverbal signals. If not attuned to these nonverbal signals, physicians could easily miss or misinterpret patient requests for information or reassurance.

A second explanation for an association between patients' sociodemographic characteristics and the medical care process is that physicians may be consciously and quite appropriately addressing the varying responses to illness that socially patterned expectations for care demand. These needs reflect the diverse attitudes, beliefs, and expectations of the groups to which the patients belong (Fox & Storms, 1981). For instance, in his classic study of ethnicity and pain, Zborowski (1952) found that patients' interpretation of pain and expectations regarding pain control varied widely across ethnic groups, and that members of these groups communicated these expectations to their physicians. In these instances, tailoring pain management effectively maximized medical care.

Finally, it is possible that physicians, like others in our society, are negatively affected by stereotypes. Physicians have generally scored about the same as nonphysicians in surveys reflecting attitudes toward the elderly or the poor (Marshal, 1981; Price, Desmond, Snyder, & Kimmel, 1988). Further, the range in physicians' political and ideological beliefs indicates a broad spectrum of response to patient groups (Waitzkin, 1985). Physicians appear to adhere to the same negative stereotypes about physically unattractive people held by most others in our society (Nordholm, 1980). Physicians' negative attitudes or the assumptions they make about a patient's personality, motivation, or level of understanding clearly have implications for the care they give.

In this chapter we will explore the extent to which the literature presents evidence of patient characteristics, such as age, gender, social class, ethnicity, and physical appearance, affecting doctor-patient communication.

AGE

It has been maintained that ageism, the system of destructive false beliefs about the elderly, is pervasive in our society and is reflected in the health context through negative physician attitudes and a general reluctance to deal with older patients (Haug, 1981; Greene et al., 1986). However, evidence of the direct manifestation of attitudes in medical practice with the elderly is sparse and somewhat contradictory.

A rare study specifically designed to compare the communication in medical visits of patients over the age of sixty-five and those forty-five years of age or younger was undertaken by Greene and associates (1986). Forty patient visits (twenty patients in each age group matched by physician, sex, and race) were audiotaped and coded for medical topics, communication content, and emotional exchange. The investigators found little evidence of blatant ageism, but did find some differences in how topics were addressed, the emotional tone of the visit, and several patterns of exchange that were related to patient age. More medical topics and fewer psychosocial issues were discussed in interviews with older patients, and further, when older patients raised psychosocial issues, doctors tended to be less responsive than when younger patients raised similar issues. Physicians were rated higher regarding the degree of questioning, information provided, and support given to younger compared to older patients. In additional analysis, the investigators report that agreement on the major goals and major medical topics discussed during the medical visit was significantly greater for younger patients and their physicians than for older patients (Greene, Adelman, Charon, & Friedmann, 1989).

In terms of the emotional tone of the visit, observers listening to audiotapes rated physician behavior as significantly less positive when with elderly patients. Physicians were less egalitarian, patient, engaged, and respectful when with older patients (Greene et al., 1986). Also concluding that visits with elderly patients may carry more tension than those of younger patients, Stewart (1983) found that physicians were less likely to engage in "tension release"—jokes and laughter—when with older patients, and that older patients were much more likely to express antagonism or defensiveness than younger patients.

There is some evidence from the investigation of nonverbal or paralinguistic qualities of interaction to suggest that communication between elderly patients and providers differs from that of younger patients. This question was explored by Caporael (1981), focusing on the use of displaced baby talk to the institutionalized elderly. Baby talk is a simplified speech pattern with distinctive paralinguistic features of high pitch and exaggerated intonation contour, usually associated with speech to young children (see Caporael, 1981, for a detailed discussion of this area). More than 22% of speech to residents in one nursing home was coded as baby talk. Further, even talk from caregivers to the elderly that was not identified as baby talk was more likely to be judged as directed toward a child than was talk between caregivers. The investigators concluded that this phenomenon was widespread and that baby talk directed toward elderly adults was not a result of fine tuning of speech to individual needs or characteristics of a particular patient, but rather a function of social stereotyping of the elderly.

The final interpretation of these findings is not straightforward. Whether these messages are perceived positively or not was also investigated. It was found that when baby talk was stripped of its context and content filtered it sounded more comforting, less irritating, and less arousing than adult talk. When rated in context, however, that is when played to judges who were themselves institutionalized elderly, preference was related to functional ability: the lower the elderly judge's functional ability, the more positively baby talk was rated (Caporael, Lukaszewski, & Culbertson, 1983).

In contrast to the findings described above, several other investigators have concluded that the elderly appear to have some advantage over younger patients in communication with physicians. For instance, Hooper and colleagues (Hooper, Comstock, Goodwin, & Goodwin, 1982) found physicians to be more courteous with elderly compared to younger patients. This effect, however, was only evident for patients over the age of seventy-four. Physicians also spent significantly more time and gave more information to patients over the age of forty. In other research, there was evidence of greater warmth directed toward the "old-old," that is, patients over the age of seventy-four (Roter, 1991), and little evidence otherwise that increasing age influences the content or effectiveness of communication (Rost & Roter, 1987). Waitzkin (1985) reported that older patients in his study appeared to receive more explanations in nontechnical and comprehensible language, and more explanations that were matched to the sophistication of the question than younger patients. It should be noted, however, that since age was positively associated with both poorer prognosis and longer acquaintance with the physician, these elements may have influenced the observed relationships with age.

In sum, older patients appear to have some advantages—they receive more communication overall, and especially more information, than younger patients. Older patients may, nonetheless, be subject to a subtle ageism, which is reflected in the tone and quality of interactions rather than directly in blatant bias or name calling (Greene et al., 1986).

GENDER

Although almost everyone is intrigued by differences in male and female behavior patterns, medical care researchers have not given this topic much attention until recently. And although a typical study will have ample numbers of male and female patients, it will not typically have ample numbers of male and female physicians—usually the physician sample is small and at least two-thirds male. Therefore, the crucial question of how physician and patient gender interact in shaping the process of care is hard to address. Nevertheless, the available literature on patient gender offers some thought-provoking findings. (Results related to physician gender are discussed in Chapter 4.)

The effects of one's gender on health care use is evident at even a young age. A study investigating the potential for children's active participation in their own health care was conducted in the late 1970s (Lewis, Lewis, Lorimer, & Palmer, 1977). The study team established a procedure within an elementary school in Los Angeles whereby children aged five through twelve were permitted to act independently of adults in seeking care from the school nurse. These children were free to leave the classroom and seek out the nurse without approval of their teacher.

The care-seeking patterns of these children were studied before initiation of the study and after two years. Before the study, boys and girls had about the same number of visits to the nurse. After two years, the care-seeking patterns of these children were virtually identical to those of adults. Children from more affluent backgrounds made more visits, and girls came more often than boys. For each visit a boy made to the nurse, girls made 1.5—virtually identical to the sex ratio for adults thirty-five to fifty-four years of age, 1.55 female visits for each male visit (Lewis et al., 1977).

In a study focusing on patient gender differences in communication, Waitzkin (1985) found that female patients were given more information than male patients, and that the information was given in a more comprehensible manner, that is, technical matters were explained or reworded in simpler language. There was also a tendency for physicians to match their response to female patients' questions in terms of technical sophistication, consequently avoiding the appearance of talking up or talking down to them (Waitzkin, 1985). In an analysis of the same data set, Wallen and associates (Wallen, Waitzkin, & Stoeckle, 1979) demonstrated that the greater amount of information directed toward women was largely in response to women's tendency to ask more questions in general and to ask more questions following the doctor's explanation.

Very similar conclusions were drawn by Pendleton and Bochner (1980) in their English study of general consultations. These investigators found that female patients were given more information than males and that this information was in answer to their more frequent questions. Our own research on one hundred routine medical visits at a large teaching hospital did not find that female patients obtained more information overall. However, they had more medical/technical jargon addressed to them and, more frequently than males, asked for explanations of these terms. In this study, female patients also gave more information of a medical nature to the doctor than male patients did—perhaps in reciprocation of receiving more technical language (Hall, Irish, Roter, Ehrlich, & Miller, 1992).

Several other investigators report that female patients receive more positive talk and more attempts to include them in discussion than males. Stewart's analysis of some 140 audiotapes of primary care practice found that physicians were more likely to express "tension release" (laughter, mainly) with female patients, and were also more inclined to ask them about their opinions or feelings (Stewart, 1983). Female patients were more likely to express tension and ask for help than were males, but male patients appeared more likely to take the initiative in exchange. For instance, males showed higher scores on a "patient-centered" cluster of behaviors, which included such patient behaviors as giving suggestions, opinions, information, and orientation to the physician, as well as more negative verbal behaviors, including disagreements and antagonisms.

A direct observational study of some 150 patient visits reported by Hooper and colleagues (Hooper et al., 1982) similarly concluded that female patients had more positive experiences with their physicians than male patients. Information giving by the physician was significantly higher and there was greater use of empathy with female compared to male patients. Physicians were also less likely to interrupt the visit by leaving the room when with female compared to male patients.

While there are studies that have failed to find any association between patient gender and studied aspects of communication (Beisecker & Beisecker, 1990), none has showed less information given to female patients. As noted by Hooper and colleagues (1982), communication differences attributable to gender may reflect sexism in medical encounters, but this may act to the advantage of female patients, who have a more informative and positive experience than is typical for male patients.

Many studies in nonmedical settings have also shown differences in male and female communication styles. It is not unreasonable to expect that these differences may also show up in how doctors and patients act toward each other. In general, the interpersonal style of women is more engaged, warm, and immediate (Hall, 1984, 1987). The sexes differ in their use of smiling, facial expressiveness, gazing, interpersonal distance, angle of facing another person, touch, and bodily gestures—with women in each case showing a behavior pattern that suggests more accessibility and friendliness. Women emit more "back channel" responses—nod, "uh-huh," "yeah," and "I see"—which serve to encourage the other's speech and show attention. Women often find it easier than men do to disclose information about themselves in conversation (Aries, 1987).

Women and men differ in their communication skills, both overall (Sarason, Sarason, Hacker, & Basham, 1985) and in terms of nonverbal communication in particular (Hall, 1984). Women decode the meanings of nonverbal cues better than men do (e.g., facial expressions, tone of voice), and also express emotions more accurately through nonverbal cues than men do.

These patterns, along with the data presented earlier on utilization patterns of the sexes and the amount of information gained from doctors, could certainly have implications for medical care. Future research may reveal that women are more savvy users of their time with doctors. Communication may be more effective in terms of factual information exchange as well as the more subtle aspects of understanding the doctor's feelings and intentions.

People also treat the sexes differently—for example, by gazing more at women than at men, and sitting or standing closer to women than to men. Together, these patterns mean that women interacting with women are the most immediate nonverbally, while men with men are the least so (Hall, 1984). Sometimes differential treatment of the sexes may reflect disrespect or disregard for one sex. In our study of one hundred internal medicine visits, physicians (who were evenly divided between males and females) used voices with a more bored, calm, and submissive tone when addressing female patients. Although the voice tone findings could indicate that physicians were tuning out female patients, an alternative interpretation is that physicians' less active and less dominant manner with females simply reflects a more low-key manner of interaction. This would be consistent with other research that finds voice tone addressed to males to be the most businesslike, condescending, and dominant (Hall & Braunwald, 1981). In our study, there were few other differences in the treatment of male versus female patients, and few differences in the patient's own behavior as a function of his or her gender.

SOCIAL CLASS

In one of the first studies of social class and culture on health, Koos (1954) found not only that recognition of serious symptoms differed among the classes but that the social evaluation of the symptoms differed. For instance, Koos found that working-class women often suffered from persistent backaches but rarely sought medical care for them. Further, these women felt that undue attention to so common a condition would inspire ridicule rather than sympathy. In contrast, women of higher social classes were much more likely to rate persistent backache as a serious symptom deserving medical attention.

A second process may also be at work. Some symptoms and social roles may be mutually supporting, that is, some symptoms may be seen as evidence of especially good or dedicated performance. For instance, in a study with graduate students, it was found that tiredness was often recorded in symptom diaries but infrequently noted as a reason for concern. For these students, fatigue meant they were working hard and was taken as an indication of doing the right thing. Consequently few students saw persistent fatigue as a reason for seeking medical help, even though they were well aware of the host of quite serious medical and psychological conditions often associated with it. Fatigue became something to be proud of, and to talk about, rather than a cause of concern (Zola, 1966).

The effect of social class on patients' presentation of themselves and their problems also has relevance for the medical treatment patients receive. Doctors talk more with patients who are higher in social class. This has been found in Florida, Massachusetts, California, England, and Scotland. We can ask how such treatment affects the patient and also what accounts for such findings. Does the higher social class patient have more to say? Does this patient not have more to say, but instead has the assertiveness to say it? Does the doctor give more opportunity for such a patient to talk, by nonverbal indications of interest and by asking more inviting questions?

It is also known that doctors give more information, in particular, to the higher-class patients, even though, when asked later, patients of different classes do not differ in how much information they say they want. Pendleton and Bochner (1980), in their English videotape study of seventy-nine general consultations, found that patients' social class was a significant predictor of how many explanations were volunteered by doctors. Physicians spontaneously offered more explanations to patients of higher-class backgrounds during visits than to other patients. The investigators suggest that physician explanations are less likely to be volunteered to patients of lower-class backgrounds because they are perceived as less interested in information and are more diffident in the asking of questions.

In an earlier Scottish study, Bain (1976) found that patients of lower-class backgrounds were less verbally active overall during medical visits than others; this was especially evident in such areas as patient presentation of their symptoms, the asking of questions, and social talk. Physicians were much more likely to give higher-class patients information regarding problem resolution and to engage in social talk with them than with lower-class patients. In further analysis of these data, Bain (1977) found that communication regarding drugs was significantly less successful with patients of lower socioeconomic backgrounds as their recall of diagnosis, drugs prescribed, and advice given regarding how often drugs should be taken and the duration of treatment was lower than other patients. Later, Bain's (1979) study in the United States, involving 22 physicians and a total of 556 patients, confirmed similar differences in the overall content of communications for patients from different socioeconomic groups. Patients with higher socioeconomic backgrounds engaged in nearly 60% more talk with the physician during the visit than patients from lower socioeconomic groups.

Work by Cartwright and others appears to support the contention that patients of lower-class backgrounds appear diffident in asking questions, not because they do not wish to know about medical matters, but rather because the social distance between themselves and their physicians discourages verbal assertiveness (Cartwright, 1967). Waitzkin (1985) attributes the paucity of direct questions by working-class patients to their sociolinguistic culture, which tends to be less verbal than that of the middle class. Because of the tendency away from direct, verbal communication, working-class patients may be communicating their desire for information in ways physicians are likely to miss. Doctors, like other members of the middle class, expect communication to be verbal and explicit; if patients have questions, doctors expect that patients will ask them. Consequently, unsolicited information is not offered and reticence is taken as an indication of disinterest.

Waitzkin's (1985) large study in the United States found that better-educated patients and patients from higher socioeconomic backgrounds received more physician time, more total explanations, and more explanations in comprehensible language than other patients. Ironically, physicians not only gave more information to higher-class patients, they also appeared to go out of their way to offer these explanations in clear, nontechnical language. Multivariate analysis of these data further demonstrated that patients' level of education was more important than social class in general in explaining information transmittal. Thus Waitzkin concludes that the educational aspect of social class determination is a particularly strong factor in doctor-patient communication.

In a similar vein, Stewart (1983) reports that better-educated patients were much more likely to receive a justification for their treatment regimens from their physicians than less educated patients. In this study, however, more information came at the price of communication offering emotional support. The better-educated patients in this study received less "solidarity" from their physicians than did those patients without some university-level training.

The opposite finding in regard to emotional support has been reported in several communication studies of pediatric visits wherein better-educated parents of patients received more emotional support than less educated parents. The classic study by Korsch and associates (Korsch, Gozzi, & Francis, 1968) of pediatric encounters in an emergency walk-in clinic found that better-educated parents of patients were more likely to express their fears and hopes to the doctor, and that they had a better chance of having these responded to or dealt with than less educated parents. Similarly, the pediatric study by Wasserman and associates (Wasserman, Inui, Barriatua, Carter, & Lippincott, 1983) found that better-educated mothers received more reassurance, encouragement, and empathy during pediatric visits than less educated mothers. Finally, in the most extensive observational study of pediatric practice, Ross and Duff (1982) observed indicators of performance quality, both technical and interpersonal, in over four hundred pediatric visits and reported that poorly educated parents received worse care on all accounts from their physicians. Also noted in this study was that low-income families did not have as consistently negative experiences as did the children of the poorly educated. Thus these authors concluded, as did Waitzkin (1985), that education has more significance for health care experience than other socioeconomic indicators.

In sum, we can say that physicians engage in more talk overall, especially more informative talk, with patients of higher as compared to lower social classes. Moreover, the evidence suggests that it is education that may play a key role in the differential communication to patients of varying socioeconomic groups. The communication advantage for the better-educated is especially evident in socioemotional support expressed during pediatric encounters.

It has long been known that poorer and less educated patients have trouble finding health care and get less of it. Now it appears that the problems of these groups are not entirely structural. They suffer poorer treatment even after they gain access to the health care system. The poor also have worse health, and although this has usually been assumed to stem from lifestyle factors such as stress or poor nutrition, or from difficulties in getting care, the possibility must also be raised that disadvantaged patients may be sicker partly because of the way in which they and their doctors communicate.

ETHNICITY

Ethnic origin and cultural background not only contribute to the definition of what symptoms are noteworthy, but also are responsible for how symptoms will be presented to the physician. A classic study of health and ethnicity (Zola, 1963) found that among patients seeking medical care from several different outpatient clinics, those of Italian rather than Irish or Anglo-Saxon descent were much more likely to be labeled as having psychiatric problems by their physicians, despite the lack of objective evidence that these problems were more frequent among them. For instance, when the doctors could not identify any specific disease to explain the patient's symptoms, which happened equally often in each of the ethnic groups, Italians almost always had their symptoms attributed to psychological problems; this almost never happened in the case of the Anglo-Saxons and Irish.

Differences were evident in how the Italians presented their chief complaints. Italians reported more pain, more symptoms overall and in more bodily locations, and more consequent dysfunction, including interference with their social and personal relations. From these findings, the investigator speculates that the Italians and Irish have ways of communicating illness that reflect different ways of handling problems within the culture itself. The Italians tend toward drama and exaggeration as a means of dissipating and coping with anxiety, whereas the Irish have a tradition in which control and denial are foremost (Barzini, 1965). This became evident in the very different ways these patients presented their symptoms to their doctors.

Similar findings were reported by Zborowski (1952) in describing ethnic variations in response to pain. Anglo-Saxon patients viewed pain in an objective and rather unemotional way, the Irish often denied pain, and Italian and Jewish patients were highly emotional and exaggerated in their pain expression. Moreover, the Italian patients sought immediate relief from pain and were satisfied as soon as the pain ceased, but the Jewish patients were more concerned about the significance of their pain for future health and resisted pain medication for fear that it would mask a significant symptom. Not only was the way in which patients presented their pain significant, but appropriate treatment was tied to this expression. Painkillers would be effective for the Italian patients, but not for the Jewish patients until reassurance about future health was also provided. Only a physician sensitive to these distinctions could appropriately recognize these needs.

A follow-up study, using the same clinics as in the Zborowski study some twenty years later (Koopman, Eisenthal, & Stoeckle, 1984), found similar differences in pain reporting between Anglos and Italians; however, the effects of culture were most evident with patients over sixty years of age. The patient's sex was also found to be an important factor in this study; pain was most likely to be reported by older female Italians and least likely to be reported by older male Anglos. For younger patients, now the second and third generation in this country, the process of acculturation had diminished the ethnic effects.

Given the correlation between social class and ethnicity in our society, it is not surprising that doctors' treatment of patients in different ethnic groups tends to parallel that for different social classes. Whites have been shown to receive care of higher technical and interpersonal quality than blacks or Hispanics receive, as well as to receive more positive talk and more information, even within the same medical practices (Hall, Roter, & Katz, 1988; Tuckett, Boulton, Olson, & Williams, 1985). One study found that blacks received fewer recommendations for open-heart surgery, although they had equal clinical need, and that of all patients who received such a recommendation, blacks had surgery less often (Maynard, Fisher, Passamani, & Pullum, 1986).

One of the few communication studies to address directly the issue of ethnicity found that physicians demonstrated better questioning and facilitating skills and more empathy skills when with Anglo-American as compared to Spanish-American patients (Hooper et al., 1982). The investigators suggest that poorer performance is particularly evident in communication skills requiring listening.

We believe that negative stereotypes of disadvantaged social groups affect the way doctors interact with these patients. We also believe this is unintentional and that doctors are only dimly aware of differences in their behavior, if at all. Like most people, doctors probably attribute any differences they do notice in their own behaviors to the character, aptitude, or needs of the other (in this case, the lower-class or minority patient). When one's own behavior can be construed as negative, a person is particularly inclined to blame it on the other. Such a process of attributing one's own behavior to causes outside of oneself greatly decreases the likelihood that doctors will recognize a connection between their own attitudes and their behavior.

OTHER PATIENT CHARACTERISTICS

Addressing the influence of physical appearance on doctor-patient communication, Hooper and associates (1982) rated the physical appearance of the patients included in their observational study. Patients who appeared rumpled, disheveled, or with dirty clothing had encounters in which the physician was less likely to use appropriate open-ended questions, to elicit details, and to allow the patient an opportunity to ask questions. Similar differences were evident in nonverbal communication, including eye contact and physician's body position, and observers' ratings of courtesy. Patients with the highest ratings on appearance—those who were "clean and pressed" in a three-piece suit or attractive dress, hair clean and neatly styled—had fewer physician-initiated interruptions during their visits than other patients. These findings are quite similar to the negative experiences reported for patients of lower socioeconomic or ethnic minority backgrounds.

Because of the difficulty in investigating the influence of patients' psychological and personality characteristics on medical visits in natural settings, an analogue study worthy of note was conducted by Gerbert (1984). In this study ninety-three physicians described their likely behavior in response to videotape vignettes. The researchers had manipulated the vignettes to depict patients in varying combinations of likability and competence. After viewing videotapes in which patients were portrayed as incompetent, the physicians indicated they would give them extra education; they would interview patients who were unlikable for psychological data; and finally, they would encourage the likable and competent patients to contact the office more often and receive more medication than other patients.

The continuum of likability in this study is reminiscent of the personality attributes of the hateful patient described by Groves (1978). The hateful patient appears to physicians as overly dependent, demanding, manipulative, rejecting, or self-destructive. Groves suggests that the negative reactions these patients evoke from their physicians should be used as clinical data to facilitate better understanding and more appropriate psychosocial management. If the findings of the analogue study can be generalized to the clinical situation, then this advice appears to be well taken by the study physicians, in that hateful patients have more psychological attention given to them. Likewise, beneficial treatment of incompetent patients in terms of increased education would appear appropriate. Thus Gerbert concludes that on the whole physicians in her study acted in their patients' best interest when confronted with negative patient attributes (Gerbert, 1984), although one might argue that the implicit label of incompetent or unlikable in itself carries negative connotations and possible negative consequences.

Though physicians will undoubtedly be uncomfortable with the suggestion that their personal liking of patients makes a difference in their care, it is probable that the medical visit, like any other interpersonal encounter, is influenced by approach and avoidance tendencies on the part of both physician and patient. Though there is not much work focusing specifically on liking, there is a great deal of indirect evidence to suggest that liking matters in medical visits.

First, whenever a study shows that doctors treat patients of different types differently, one must ask whether stereotypes are translating into degrees of liking and disliking for whole categories of patients. Research that asks physicians for their attitudes and beliefs about various groups such as male and female patients, difficult versus easy patients, physically attractive versus unattractive patients, and patients of different social classes does suggest that physicians' attitudes vary across such groups (Bernstein & Kane, 1981; Smith & Zimny, 1988; Nordholm, 1980; Dungal, 1978; Leiderman & Grisso, 1985; Biener, 1983).

Second, contrary to the stereotype of physicians as consistent and neutral in their interpersonal behaviors, there is much evidence that the affective quality of interactions varies a great deal, and furthermore that the level of affect (anger, for example) displayed by the patient is reflected back in the physician's nonverbal behavior and vice versa (Hall, Roter, & Rand, 1981). Liking could certainly be playing a role in establishing the affective tone of the interaction.

Third, there is a small amount of research that directly assesses liking and its possible impact. Both Like and Zyzanski (1987) and Hall, Epstein, DeCiantis, and McNeil (1993) asked physicians to rate their liking for specific patients, by name. The physician's liking of the patient and the patient's satisfaction with his or her medical care were significantly related in both studies. More sensitive research designs will be needed to determine the causal patterns inherent in this correlation. Does the physician's liking of the patient cause the patient to be satisfied, and if so, does this come about as a simple reaction to warm versus cool nonverbal signals? Or does the physician's liking translate into different quality of care provided—more earnest discussion of issues, more vigilant monitoring of signs and side effects, and so forth? Alternatively, does the patient's level of satisfaction cause the patient to behave in a more or less likable way, thus producing corresponding variations in the physician's liking of the patient? Surely the satisfaction-liking spiral could be playing an extremely important role in determining both the patient's and the doctor's commitment to each other and to the patient's well-being.

The study by Hall and colleagues (1993) also related other patient characteristics to physicians' liking of patients. Male patients were more liked, overall, than were female patients by the seventeen (predominantly male) physicians in the sample. In a larger physician sample, one could determine whether the physician's gender also matters here—perhaps physicians tend to like patients of their own gender the most. If it is generally the case that male patients are liked more, this could have implications for the quality of exchange and for patient care outcomes. For instance, the finding that females received less diagnostic testing for coronary disease, even when their condition was equivalent to that of the males in the sample (Tobin, Wassertheil-Smoller, Wexler, Steingart, Budner, Lense, & Wachspress, 1987), may signal preferential treatment for males as well as different communication patterns with male versus female patients.

Hall et al. (1993) also found that physicians liked their healthier patients more than their less healthy ones, whether health was defined in terms of social, emotional, or functional criteria, or was rated overall by the patient, and even when standard patient sociodemographic characteristics were controlled for. We believe this to be a disturbing result and one that may come as a surprise to physicians, who probably believe they find the more challenging cases to be most stimulating and rewarding. Indeed, this may be true in certain cases, but the prevailing fact of routine medical practice is that many serious medical conditions are chronic (especially in the elderly population used in this study), and therefore do not offer the rewards of a cure nor the variety and excitement of an acute condition. Patients with chronic conditions may also cease acting very appreciative since they are not getting cured and indeed may be on a downward slide. Finally, patients who do not feel good are likely to be grumpy, unresponsive, and possibly unwashed or unkempt; patients whose distress is of an emotional nature may be particularly erratic or unrewarding in interpersonal interaction. Thus, it is not too surprising if physicians have more feelings of liking for their patients in better condition.

However understandable a physician's reaction may be, the implications could of course be great. One common finding from research on patient satisfaction is that sicker and more distressed patients are less satisfied with their care, as summarized by Pascoe (1983) and Hall, Feldstein, Fretwell, Rowe, and Epstein (1990). Although this result could stem from the generally negative outlook likely to be held by a person in physical or mental distress, it could also stem from negative cues given off unconsciously by the physician.

There appears to be evidence for all three earlier hypothesized mechanisms by which patient characteristics may affect doctor-patient communication. There may be unintended violations of universalism due to miscommunication, with patients from lower socioeconomic backgrounds not making their desire for information clear to physicians, as suggested by Waitzkin (1985); divergent response tendencies of patients, for instance more asking of questions by female patients, leading to more information directed toward female compared with male patients; and, finally, perhaps there are unconscious violations of a universalistic orientation through stereotypes, dislike, and prejudice, as in interaction with unlikable or "difficult" patients.

There are certainly differences in doctor-patient communication that may be attributable to differences in such patient characteristics as sex, age, race, educational level, and social class. What is not clear from the body of literature reviewed is whether these distinctions are uniformly negative in their effect on patient care. In regard to gender, for instance, Hooper et al. (1982) suggest that in contrast to the widely publicized view that medical care is given in a way that disparages or discriminates against women, sexism may work in favor of better medical care for female patients. This is consistent with utilization studies that have established that females receive more services than males, including return visits, tests, and prescriptions (Verbrugge & Steiner, 1981; Weisman & Teitelbaum, 1989). Beneficial treatment for the elderly is less clear; older patients may receive more information than others but it may be communicated in a manner reflective of subtle ageism, undermining their effectiveness as participants in medical exchanges. Less conflicting evidence has been found in regard to the experience of patients from lower social class backgrounds, minorities, and the poorly educated—these patients have more negative health experiences than others.

In their careful analysis, Hooper and colleagues (1982) determined that the four patient characteristics they studied—age, sex, physical appearance, and ethnic origin—acted independently in influencing physician behavior. Waitzkin (1985), however, failed to find any independent contribution of sex or social class to variation in physicians' information-giving behavior, so that only patients' age and educational level appeared in these analyses to be significant predictors of differential communication.

We do not claim that communication deficiencies are entirely a matter of doctors' attitudes and have nothing to do with how different kinds of patients behave. A highly verbal, college-educated patient will certainly make different demands than an immigrant with an elementary school education. But because these patients' psychological and physical needs may be exactly the same, doctors cannot base their responses entirely on the patient's initiatives. Unfortunately, for a doctor to see past immediate demands and try to fathom unexpressed patient agendas may require more patience and sensitivity than many harried doctors, with their minimal training in interpersonal skills, are willing to muster.

Although the social class, education, and ethnicity of patients cannot be changed, providers' behaviors might change if both they and their patients became more aware of how these characteristics intrude into the supposedly neutral provision of medical care. This would be a first step toward reducing their impact.

REFERENCES

Aries, E. (1987). Gender and communication. In Shaver, P., & Hendrick, C. (Eds.), *Review of personality and social psychology*, vol. 7. Newbury Park, Calif.: Sage Publications.

Bain, D. J. (1976). Doctor-patient communication in general practice consultations. *Medical Education, 10*, 125–131.

Bain, D. J. (1977). Patient knowledge and the content of the consultation in general practice. *Medical Education, 11*, 347–350.

Bain, D. J. (1979). The content of physician/patient communication in family practice. *Journal of Family Practice, 8*, 745–753.

Barzini, L. (1965). *The Italians*. New York: Bantam Press.

Beisecker, A. E., & Beisecker, T. D. (1990). Patient information-seeking behaviors when communicating with doctors. *Medical Care, 28*, 19–28.

Bernstein, B., & Kane, R. (1981). Physicians' attitudes toward female patients. *Medical Care, 19*, 600–608.

Biener, L. (1983). Perceptions of patients by emergency room staff: Substance-abusers versus non-substance-abusers. *Journal of Health and Social Behavior, 24*, 264–275.

Caporael, L. R. (1981). The paralanguage of caregiving: Baby talk to the institutionalized aged. *Journal of Personality and Social Psychology, 40*, 876–884.

Caporael, L. R., Lukaszewski, M. P., & Culbertson, G. H. (1983). Secondary baby talk: Judgments by institutionalized elderly and their caregivers. *Journal of Personality and Social Psychology, 44*, 746–756.

Cartwright, A. (1967). *Patients and their doctors*. London: Routledge & Kegan Paul.

Dungal, L. (1978). Physicians' responses to patients: A study of factors involved in the office interview. *Journal of Family Practice, 6*, 1065–1073.

Fox, J. G., & Storms, D. M. (1981). A different approach to sociodemographic predictors of satisfaction with health care. *Social Science & Medicine, 15A*, 557–564.

Gerbert, B. (1984). Perceived likeability and competence of simulated patients: Influence on physicians' management plans. *Social Science & Medicine, 18*, 1053–1060.

Greene, M. G., Adelman, R. D., Charon, R., & Friedmann, E. (1989). Concordance between physicians and their older and younger patients in the primary care medical encounter. *The Gerontologist, 29,* 808–813.

Greene, M. G., Adelman, R., Charon, R., & Hoffman, S. (1986). Ageism in the medical encounter: An exploratory study of the language and behavior of doctors with their old and young patients. *Language and Communication, 6,* 113–124.

Groves, J. E. (1978). Taking care of the hateful patient. *New England Journal of Medicine, 298,* 883–887.

Hall, J. A. (1984). *Nonverbal sex differences: Communication accuracy and expressive style.* Baltimore: Johns Hopkins University Press.

Hall, J. A. (1987). On explaining gender differences: The case of nonverbal communication. In Shaver, P., & Hendrick, C. (Eds.), *Review of Personality and Social Psychology,* vol. 7. Newbury Park, Calif.: Sage Publications.

Hall, J. A., & Braunwald, K. G. (1981). Gender cues in conversations. *Journal of Personality and Social Psychology, 40,* 99–110.

Hall, J. A., Epstein, A. M., DeCiantis, M. L., & McNeil, B. J. (1993). Physicians' liking for their patients: More evidence for the role of affect in medical care. *Health Psychology,* forthcoming.

Hall, J. A., Feldstein, M., Fretwell, M. D., Rowe, J. W., & Epstein, A. M. (1990). Older patients' health status and satisfaction with medical care in an HMO population. *Medical Care, 28,* 261–270.

Hall, J. A., Irish, J. T., Roter, D. L., Ehrlich, C. M., & Miller, L. H. (1992). Gender in medical encounters: An analysis of physicians' and patients' communication behaviors. Unpublished manuscript.

Hall, J. A., Roter, D. L., & Katz, N. R. (1988). Meta-analysis of correlates of provider behavior in medical encounters. *Medical Care, 26,* 657–675.

Hall, J. A., Roter, D. L., & Rand, C. S. (1981). Communication of affect between patient and physician. *Journal of Health and Social Behavior, 22,* 18–30.

Haug, M. R. (Ed.) (1981). *Elderly patients and their doctors.* New York: Springer Publishing.

Hooper, E. M., Comstock, L. M., Goodwin, J. M., & Goodwin, J. S. (1982). Patient characteristics that influence physician behavior. *Medical Care, 20,* 630–638.

Koopman, C. S., Eisenthal, S., & Stoeckle, J. (1984). Ethnicity in the reported pain, emotional distress and requests of medical outpatients. *Social Science & Medicine, 6,* 487–490.

Koos, E. L. (1954). *The health of Regionville.* New York: Columbia University Press.

Korsch, B. M., Gozzi, E. K., & Francis, V. (1968). Gaps in doctor-patient communication. *Pediatrics, 42,* 855–871.

Leiderman, D. B., & Grisso, J. (1985). The GOMER phenomenon. *Journal of Health and Social Behavior, 26,* 222–232.

Lewis, C. E., Lewis, M. A., Lorimer, A., & Palmer, B. B. (1977). Child-initiated care: The use of school nursing services by children in an "adult-free" system. *Pediatrics, 60,* 499–507.

Like, R., & Zyzanski, S. J. (1987). Patient satisfaction and the clinical encounter: Social psychological determinants. *Social Science & Medicine, 24*, 351–357.

Marshal, V.W. (1981). Physician characteristics and relationships with older patients. In Haug, M. R. (Ed.), *Elderly patients and their doctors*. New York: Springer Publishing.

Maynard, C. L., Fisher, D., Passamani, E. R., & Pullum, T. (1986). Blacks in the Coronary Artery Surgery Study (CASS): Race and clinical decision making. *American Journal of Public Health, 76*, 1446–1448.

Nordholm, L. A. (1980). Beautiful patients are good patients: Evidence for the physical attractiveness stereotype in first impressions of patients. *Social Science & Medicine, 14A*, 81–83.

Parsons, T. (1951). *The social system*. Glencoe, Ill.: The Free Press.

Pascoe, G. C. (1983). Patient satisfaction in primary health care: A literature review and analysis. *Evaluation and Program Planning, 6*, 185–210.

Pendleton, D. A., & Bochner, S. (1980). The communication of medical information in general practice consultations as a function of patients' social class. *Social Science & Medicine, 14A*, 669–673.

Price, J. H., Desmond, S. M., Snyder, F. F., & Kimmel, S. R. (1988). Perceptions of family practice residents regarding health care and poor patients. *Journal of Family Practice, 27*, 615–621.

Ross, C. R., & Duff, R. S. (1982). Returning to the doctor: The effects of client characteristics, type of practice, and experiences with care. *Journal of Health and Social Behavior, 23*, 119–131.

Rost, K., & Roter, D. (1987). Predictors of recall of medication regimens and recommendations for lifestyle change in elderly patients. *The Gerontologist, 27*, 510–515.

Roter, D. (1991). Elderly patient-physician communication: A descriptive study of content and affect during the medical encounter. *Advances in Health Education, 3*, 15–23.

Roter, D. L., Hall, J. A., & Katz, N. R. (1988). Patient-physician communication: A descriptive review of the literature. *Patient Education and Counseling, 12*, 99–119.

Sarason, B. R., Sarason, I. G., Hacker, T. A., & Basham, R. B. (1985). Concomitants of social support: Social skills, physical attractiveness, and gender. *Journal of Personality and Social Psychology, 49*, 469–480.

Smith, R. C., & Zimny, G. H. (1988). Physicians' emotional reactions to patients. *Psychosomatics, 29*, 392–397.

Stewart, M. (1983). Patient characteristics which are related to the doctor-patient interaction. *Family Practice, 1*, 30–35.

Tobin, J. N., Wassertheil-Smoller, S., Wexler, J. P., Steingart, R. M., Budner, N., Lense, L., & Wachspress, J. (1987). Sex bias in considering coronary bypass surgery. *Annals of Internal Medicine, 107*, 19–25.

Tuckett, D., Boulton, M., Olson, C., & Williams, A. (1985). *Meetings between experts*. New York: Tavistock Publications.

Verbrugge, L. M., & Steiner, R. P. (1981). Physician treatment of men and women patients: Sex bias or appropriate care? *Medical Care, 19*, 609–632.

Waitzkin, H. (1985). Information giving in medical care. *Journal of Health and Social Behavior, 26*, 81–101.

Wallen, J., Waitzkin, H., & Stoeckle, J. D. (1979). Physician stereotypes about female health and illness. *Women & Health, 4*, 135–146.

Wasserman, R. C., Inui, T. S., Barriatua, R. D., Carter, W. B., & Lippincott, P. (1983). Responsiveness to maternal concern in preventive child health visits: An analysis of clinician-parent interactions. *Developmental and Behavioral Pediatrics, 4*, 171–176.

Weisman, C. S., & Teitelbaum, M. A. (1989). Women and health care communication. *Patient Education and Counseling, 13*, 183–199.

Zborowski, M. (1952). Cultural components in responses to pain. *Journal of Social Issues, 4*, 16–30.

Zola, I. K. (1963). Problems of communication, diagnosis, and patient care: The interplay of patient, physician and clinic organization. *Journal of Medical Education, 38*, 829–838.

Zola, I. K. (1966). Culture and symptoms: An analysis of patients' presenting complaints. *American Sociological Review, 31*, 615–630.

4

The Influence of Physician Characteristics on Communication between the Doctor and the Patient

Who the doctor is—his or her profile in terms of sociodemographic background, culture, and personality, as well as the medical training experience—has relevance for how patients are treated and the kind of medicine that will be practiced.

Some people are more likely to become doctors than others. The sociodemographic profile that has traditionally characterized the medical profession is disproportionately male, white, and upper-middle-class (Mechanic, 1978). Efforts to diversify medical school enrollment since the 1960s have been somewhat successful, but only in relative terms. The most dramatic change from the 1960s to the 1980s has been a sevenfold increase, from 5% to 37%, in women entering medical school (Jonas & Etzel, 1988). Changes in other aspects of the demographic profile, however, have been more modest. Black enrollees in medical school make up about 5% of the total, with all other minorities adding another 5% (Jonas & Etzel, 1988).

Less attention has been paid in recent years to changes in the middle-class profile of medical students. However, there is little to suggest that the strong bias toward enrollment of students from the higher socioeconomic classes has changed. As parental income increases, there is a consistent increase in the percentage of students who apply to medical school and those who are accepted (Rosengren, 1980). Inasmuch as the debt burden continues to grow exponentially for medical students, from $19,697 in 1981 to an average of $33,499 in 1987 (Tudor, 1988), and as federal assistance continues to decline, it is unlikely that there will be major changes in the class structure of medicine. Considering the economic ramifications of medical school attendance, it is not surprising that the major changes have not been in social class but in gender; it appears that the daughters of the middle and upper middle classes are joining their brothers in medical school in greater numbers.

The pathway by which students arrive at a decision to become doctors also appears to reinforce the connection between the middle classes and medicine. Studying about 750 medical students, Rogoff (1957) found that half said they first considered becoming a doctor in their early teens and even younger. An impressive number of these students made their decision to enter medicine so early that the author characterized them as "born with a stethoscope in their ear." The earlier the decision to become a doctor was made, the more committed the youngster appeared to be; 83% of the medical students who made up their minds to be doctors before they were fourteen never gave serious thought to another occupation. Furthermore, the early deciders were more likely to feel that medicine was "the only career that could really satisfy them" (Rogoff, 1957).

Early decision making is especially true for children of physicians. The sons and daughters of doctors were almost twice as likely as those without a medical relative to have considered medicine as their future career before the teenage years (Rogoff, 1957). Indeed, more than 11% of medical school applicants list their father's occupation as physician (Rosengren, 1980). The strong evidence of intergenerational links in medicine is related in some measure to the very early socialization of children in medical households to aspire to medical careers, as well as the help, both material and emotional, their families are likely to give them (Hall, 1948). Many of the medical students in these studies credit their families with support and encouragement for their medical aspirations. While indications are that the early choice pattern of the mid-1950s is changing, with more late deciders than previously, the decision is still an early one compared to the time of choice among many other occupations (Kurtz & Chalfant, 1991).

The bias toward the middle class is not only in terms of socioeconomic status, but in terms of middle-class values and the middle-class work ethic. The kind of student who takes notes well and who studies and works obediently, irrespective of interest in the material, is favored by medical schools—and these students are largely from the middle class (Kurtz & Chalfant, 1991). Further, while medical students place high value on their ability to work with people and be helpful to others, they also emphasize the value of the income and prestige connected with their occupation, as well as its promise of independence and autonomy (Mechanic, 1978). All of these values, Mechanic notes, are reflective of the student's middle-class background and aspirations, which are also reflected in a basically conservative political orientation.

This is not to imply that young physicians are not idealistic. Most investigators agree that idealism is high upon entering medical school. There is no agreement, however, on what happens from then on. Several investigators have suggested that youthful idealism matures to a more reality-based vision of medicine, but one that remains basically idealistic (Kurtz & Chalfant, 1991). Some have suggested that the idealism with which students come to medicine is suspended during the training period, but resumes once schooling is complete (Light, 1975). None of these investigators credits the medical training process with inspiring or furthering anything that could be considered even close to idealism or humanism.

There are several ways of considering the significance of the physician's personal characteristics and training experience for the practice of medicine. First, while physicians obviously vary on sociodemographic and other characteristics, it is not clear that this variation will affect performance with patients in any obvious way. One might argue both sides: on the one hand, medical education is so strong a socializing process that it could act to equalize any differences in the effect of personal characteristics of those undergoing medical training. For example, one's political or social class biases may give way under the pressures of training such that all physicians adopt a "physician-appropriate" attitude. On the other hand, cultural beliefs and attitudes evolve over an entire lifetime and are likely to resist change in adulthood, even by such a total institution as medical school. A third possibility is that those who choose to enter medicine select themselves in such a way that there is no real difference in social traits even before medical education begins, despite variation in gender, ethnic background, or class origin.

This chapter will explore three classes of individual characteristics of the physician that can potentially affect how doctors talk with their patients. These include: (1) sociodemographic characteristics, (2) general attitudes and personality orientation, and (3) the nature of the medical training experience.

SOCIODEMOGRAPHIC CHARACTERISTICS OF THE PHYSICIAN

Gender

Although there are few direct observational studies that address physician gender issues in doctor-patient communication, it is known that visits with male and female physicians differ in terms of time spent with patients. Nationwide data from the National Ambulatory Medical Care Survey (NAMCS), reflecting office-based visits, found that female physicians spend

Table 4.1

Time Spent (in Minutes) with Male and Female Physicians

	SEX OF PATIENT		
	BOTH	FEMALE	MALE
SEX OF PHYSICIAN			
FEMALE			
General and Family Practice	17.6	18.3	15.7
Internal Medicine	23.5	24.4	20.4
MALE			
General and Family Practice	12.7	12.8	12.5
Internal Medicine	18.7	18.5	19.0

Adapted from Cypress, 1980, p. 15.

more time with patients than do male physicians (Cypress, 1980). For instance, as displayed in Table 4.1, in internal medicine and general and family practice, male physicians averaged almost five minutes less per patient than female physicians. Female physicians spent almost six minutes more with female patients than did male physicians with their female patients.

Since the NAMCS data are questionnaire-based rather than observational reports, one does not know how visits with male and female physicians might differ in regard to the communication content or process. One way in which the visits may differ is in the expression of empathy: the strongest physician-patient bonds may be formed in female same-sex dyads. Scully (1980) found that female residents in obstetrics-gynecology expressed more empathy than males with their female patients. Others have also found that female pediatric residents expressed significantly more statements of empathy to mothers during initial infant visits than did their male colleagues (Wasserman, Inui, Barriatua, Carter, & Lippincott, 1984).

We can speculate on what goes on in the doctor-patient relationship from a large body of research on male and female social behavior in general. This general literature usually finds women to be more empathic, more socially skilled, more equalizing of status differences, and more "immediate" in their nonverbal behavior—that is, they make more attentive and warmer use of smiles, gazes, distance, and touch. Moreover, women with women have the highest levels of eye contact, the closest interpersonal distances, and the most touching, and men with men have the lowest (Hall, 1984). Logically, a prediction that would fit with the general literature is that the highest levels of empathic and positive behaviors occur when both doctor and patient are female, and the lowest levels occur when both are male. We would also predict that revelation of personal material—the psychosocial problems that often underlie, or stem from, illness—would be enhanced in the more empathic, female pairs.

Indeed, female physicians in the NAMCS survey provided psychotherapy or therapeutic listening as a service to their primary care patients more often than did male physicians. Particularly for female physicians in practice for several years, and over the age of thirty-five, the rate of therapeutic listening was more than double that for male physicians of the same age (Cypress, 1980).

A recent study of sex differences in medical encounters explored these questions (Roter, Lipkin, & Korsgaard, 1991). A total of 537 medical visits were audiotaped for this study—104 of the visits were with the study's 26 female physicians and 61 were same-sex female visits; 433 visits were with the study's 101 male physicians and 185 were same-sex male visits.

The findings were consistent with those of the NAMCS survey. Female physicians in the study spent several minutes more with their patients, especially female patients, than did their male colleagues. Furthermore, it was talk during the early history-taking segment that accounted for much of the difference in length of the medical visits. Much of this extra talk by female physicians fell in particular categories of interaction. Female physicians engaged in significantly more positive talk, partnership building, question asking, and information giving.

Female doctors did not do all the talking in the visits—indeed, when with female physicians, both male and female patients talked more than with male physicians. Patients engaged in significantly more positive talk, more partnership talk, and were more likely to ask questions, give substantially more biomedical information, and engage in almost twice as much psychosocial talk when with female rather than male physicians.

It was striking that the differences evident in the content of the visit were most marked during the history-taking segment. These differences may indicate that female physicians are more attuned to early visit negotiation and are more patient-centered in their interviewing styles than males. The large differences in patient talk with female physicians, particularly the high frequency of psychosocial talk and partnership building, also suggest that these visits are more patient-centered, for both male and female patients. These results are consistent with a study that asked male and female physicians how much they liked individual patients. Perhaps not surprisingly, female physicians liked their patients more (Hall, Epstein, DeCiantis, & McNeil, 1993).

Social Class Origin

As discussed earlier, medicine is practiced largely by members of the middle class, and reflects middle-class ethics in terms of hard work, delayed gratification, economic independence, and autonomy (Mechanic, 1974). Medicine is also a vehicle of social mobility, but only for those who have demonstrated mastery of middle-class values through academic performance (Kurtz & Chalfant, 1991).

One effect of social class origin on the way physicians relate to patients is in terms of class-based communication styles. Several studies have demonstrated sociolinguistic differences among members of varying social classes. Reviewed by Waitzkin and Waterman (1974), the evidence suggests that there are indeed social-class differences in linguistic skills. Most prominent is a tendency for middle-class subjects to be verbally explicit, while working-class subjects tend to communicate more implicitly, through nonverbal signals. While most consideration of the consequences of these linguistic differences has been in terms of patients' communication, it is also possible that social-class background relates to differences in physicians' communication. These differences might act to enhance communication between physicians of lower social class origin with patients of similar backgrounds, or impede the ability of physicians from poorer backgrounds to communicate with patients of higher social classes (Waitzkin & Waterman, 1974).

While not well studied, this issue has been explored. Physicians' social class background, as measured by their fathers' occupations and the physician's style of communication, was studied in audiotapes of 34 doctors in 336 medical visits (Waitzkin, 1985). Doctors from upper-class or upper-middle-class backgrounds, compared with those from working-class backgrounds, tended to spend more time informing their patients, giving more explanations, and providing responses that were at the same technical level as the questions asked. The study concluded: "Orientation to verbal behavior may be a class-linked phenomenon which affects doctors as well as patients. Thus, doctors from working-class backgrounds may differ in their verbal behavior from doctors who come from a higher class position" (Waitzkin, 1985, p. 92).

Another example of the evidence of social background affecting physicians' styles of practice is found in the classic study of psychiatrists in New Haven, Connecticut, by Hollingshead and Redlich (1958). The social background of the thirty psychiatrists in the study was strongly associated with how they related to patients and their therapeutic orientation. Therapeutic orientation was found to fall within two distinct approaches to the treatment of patients. The first approach was analytic and psychological in orientation, with an emphasis on patient insight and as little physician-directiveness as possible. These psychiatrists were almost passive in relation to management of their patients and almost never performed physical or neurological examinations. The second approach was much more active and biomedical in nature. These psychiatrists were very directive in their therapy, often combining suggestions and advice with medical procedures, drugs, and neurological and physical tests.

There were marked differences in the social and cultural backgrounds of the psychiatrists in these two treatment approach groups. As a group, the analytic psychiatrists had moved upward much farther in the class structure than the directive group. Almost three-quarters of the analytic group, compared with 42% of the directive group, had moved upward one or more classes from the positions occupied by their fathers (Hollingshead & Redlich, 1958). The investigators found that the number of generations the psychiatrist's family had been in the United States was also linked to his or her theoretical orientation. Only 8% of the analytically oriented group were from old American stock, whereas 44% of the directive group were from that background. In contrast, 58% of the analytic group were first- and second-generation Americans compared with 38% of the other group.

Hollingshead and Redlich speculate about the analytic psychiatrists that "like all phenomenal upward mobile persons, those who have achieved their present class positions largely through their own efforts and abilities have passed through a social, possibly also psychological, transformation" (Hollingshead & Redlich, 1958, p. 165), which accounts for their practice style. While not specifically studied, it is interesting to speculate that the patient orientations described by Hollingshead and Redlich may also apply to primary care physicians and their tendency to relate to patients in a more or less directive manner.

Relevant to this point are the findings from a large survey of physicians (Haug & Lavin, 1983), which found that those who rose to the middle class reported greater attitudinal acceptance and behavioral accommodation to consumerist-type patient challenges than those who originally came from upper-class and upper-middle-class backgrounds. This may reflect a more directive and "take charge" orientation among physicians from higher social class origins than among those who are upwardly mobile. Haug and Lavin (1983) note that these findings are contrary to the theory that the upwardly mobile are more conforming to traditional norms.

ATTITUDES AND PERSONALITY

Political Ideology

Physicians hold views across the entire political spectrum. Nevertheless, the majority of physicians describe themselves as politically conservative and identify with the Republican party (Mechanic, 1974). In fact, it appears that most students who enter medical school are politically conservative and that this outlook is reinforced in the process of medical education (Coe, 1970). Liberal physicians and medical students appear to be the exception rather than the rule. As in other walks of life, "the ideology of physicians depends on background characteristics, the nature of their work, and their self-interest. In general physicians who tend to support social reform are those who appear to have the least to lose from it" (Mechanic, 1978, p. 399).

Mechanic found a practical consequence of political orientation in the conduct of medical practice. More liberal doctors saw fewer patients per day with a more limited scope of practice. These doctors had lower incomes and were more likely to believe that physicians have a responsibility to advise and care for the psychological problems of patients (Mechanic, 1974). How political orientation may affect the doctor-patient dynamic in actual medical encounters was investigated by Waitzkin (1985). It was found that more liberal political ideology was associated with how doctors conveyed information. Liberal doctors tended to give more explanations overall, and more explanations in understandable language, than other doctors. In a similar vein, physicians found to have lower personal needs for power gave more information to their patients (Waitzkin, 1985).

Age also appears to be a relevant issue in terms of physicians' attitudes. In one study, physicians under the age of thirty-five were nearly twice as likely as those sixty-five and over (43% versus 24%) to express attitudes consistent with a consumerist perspective (Haug & Lavin, 1983). These differences were even more marked in regard to having actually accommodated a patient request. In this case there was a fivefold difference: 57% of the younger physicians, compared to only 12% of the older physicians, reported that they had actually accommodated a consumerist patient request (Haug & Lavin, 1983).

In a similar vein, Linn and Lewis concluded from their survey of some five hundred community-based, primary care physicians in the Los Angeles area that young physicians had more positive attitudes toward patient self-care than those over the age of forty-six (Linn & Lewis, 1979).

Practice characteristics also appear to be associated with political orientation (Mechanic, 1974; Linn & Lewis, 1979). Studying a national sample of primary care physicians, Mechanic found that physicians' political views were highly correlated with the way they view the organization and delivery of medical care. Office-based, solo practitioners were more conservative than physicians in groups or in hospital-based practice, while doctors in prepaid practice and academic medicine were most likely to hold liberal political views.

The organization of medical care delivery has relevance for variation in practice patterns and, consequently, for the doctor-patient relationship. Freidson describes two types of medical practice: client-dependent and colleague-dependent (Freidson, 1970a). The client-dependent form is characterized by being wholly dependent on clients for economic survival. In order for the physician to stay in practice—to stay in business—he or she must offer services with an eye to patient demand and patients' standards and criteria of evaluation. The other form, colleague-dependent practice, relies on other professionals or organizations for client referrals. In order to survive economically, the physician must respond to collegial standards of practice rather than patient demand.

Solo practitioners and those in small group practices—including general practitioners and some internists, pediatricians, ophthalmologists, and gynecologists—are good examples of the client-dependent type. The goodwill and word-of-mouth reputation established by satisfied patients ensures a successful practice. The implication for communication and the doctor-patient relationship is that these physicians will be more responsive to patient demands for information, or for clinical services such as tests or prescriptions.

Representing the opposite extreme, such medical specialties as pathology, anesthesiology, and radiology are almost completely dependent upon colleague referrals and have little need for client-oriented techniques and "bedside manners." Bureaucratic organizations such as HMOs (health maintenance organizations), hospitals, and clinics also represent colleague-driven types, with less client responsiveness than other forms of practice (Freidson, 1970a).

Because of the patient-dependent nature of fee-for-service practice, Mechanic maintains, this form is more personalized and responsive than the prepaid group practice. The latter, because of its bureaucratic nature, is said to encourage a more assembly-line, less personal, type of practice, with physician responsiveness to the organization superseding responsiveness to the patient (Mechanic, 1974). This is especially evident when the bureaucracy's need to cut costs places the physician in a gatekeeper role, controlling access to services and thereby preventing overutilization, which is considered an abuse of the system. Indeed, there are lower rates for surgery, hospitalization, and testing in HMOs than in hospital-based or fee-for-service medical practice (Eisenberg, 1986).

Another characteristic of the prepaid practice is the contractual nature of the arrangement and the conversion of patients into bureaucratic clients. "Clients did not, like customers, threaten to take their business elsewhere; they demanded their rights under their contract and threatened bureaucratic trouble" (Freidson, 1975, p. 52). The threat of recourse to the HMO administrator or other institutional framework gives patients the additional bargaining power of a third party ally with weapons of paperwork and red tape. This potential weapon may afford patients influence even above that held by fee-paying patients seeing doctors in private practice.

An awareness of and accommodation to the bureaucratic client may explain the finding that physicians in prepaid practice were more responsive to consumerist patient demands than fee-for-service physicians (Haug & Lavin, 1983). Two-thirds of the doctors in prepaid settings reported some form of accommodation to patient demand, in contrast to 15% by fee-for-service practitioners. Again, Linn and Lewis similarly reported from their survey that physicians who were employed in a group practice or clinic were more likely to hold favorable attitudes toward patient self-care than those engaged in solo medical practice (Linn & Lewis, 1979).

Physician Personality Characteristics

In several studies, physician personality has been related to medical practice styles. The Myers-Briggs Type Inventory (MBTI) has been an especially popular measure of personality in these studies. The MBTI is an assessment inventory based on Jung's theory of personality, which assesses an individual's preferences in four areas along a continuum: perceiving (sensing—intuition), with sensing types perceiving the immediate facts of their experiences while intuitive types focus on possibilities and meanings; deciding (thinking—feeling), with thinking types making decisions impersonally and objectively while feeling types make more subjective and personal decisions; orientation (extroversion—introversion), with extroverts tending toward actions and objects while introverts tend toward concepts and ideas; and coping (judging—perception), with judging types tending toward a planned and orderly manner while perceiving types are more spontaneous and flexible (Ornstein, Markert, Johnson, Rust, & Afrin, 1988).

The MBTI has been related to test-ordering behaviors of physicians. Test ordering is a particular area of interest, not only because of the costs involved, but also because it reflects differential attitudes toward technology and uncertainty—both issues with implications for the way the doctor is likely to communicate with patients. Investigators found that introverted and intuitive physicians ordered more laboratory tests for their hypertensive patients than did their more extroverted and sensing colleagues (Ornstein et al., 1988). Fifty-three physicians who completed a program in family medicine were monitored over a three-year period to confirm preliminary observations made by the investigators. The extroversion-introversion and sensing-intuition scale scores of the physicians were both significant predictors. Introversion and intuition were positively associated with test ordering. Furthermore, personality was a more significant predictor of whether the physician ordered a test than any of the other aspects studied, including a variety of patient sociodemographic, utilization, and physical status variables.

The authors suggest that the positive associations between introversion and intuition with test ordering may be explained in the following manner. Introverts, in contrast to extroverts, are oriented toward the inner world of concepts and ideas, and are likely drawn to activities requiring sustained attention. Laboratory test ordering and follow-up can be considered such an activity. In a similar vein, intuitive individuals are more likely to operate within the realm of the imagination, are less likely to trust their sense of observation, and consequently may feel the need for additional data and reliance on impersonal analysis of possibilities.

The implications of these personality types for patterns of communication with patients are many. One might speculate that introverted and intuitive physicians, in relying heavily on tests for decision-making data, ignore the potential diagnostic clues their patients may offer. They may be using tests in lieu of talking with patients, preferring the more objective information provided through tests and other experts to the sometimes confusing thread of a patient's story of his or her illness experience.

We do know that some medical specialties attract particular kinds of personalities and values. For instance, Mechanic has characterized the personality type of several specialists:

The image of the internist is that of the intellectual problem solver, while the surgeon is seen as more aggressive and active. The family practitioner, in contrast, tends to be less conceptual and more gregarious than the internist. Psychiatry draws physicians who are abstract and playful about ideas, while surgeons tend to be more concrete and moralistic. Psychiatrists tend to be high on Machiavellianism, while surgeons tend to be low. (Mechanic, 1978, p. 382)

Physicians also vary in the interpersonal skills they bring to the medical encounter. Considering that doctoring usually involves interpersonal communication, and that patients have feelings, needs, and agendas pertinent to their medical problems, it stands to reason that communication skills play an important role in medical care. Research on physicians has focused on two specific skills: skill in expressing emotions via nonverbal cues (such as face or voice tone), and skill in decoding or recognizing others' nonverbal expressions. These skills can be reliably measured and are enduring qualities of a person. A large amount of research not pertaining specifically to physicians has demonstrated that these skills are important in marital, social, clinical, and other professional settings (for example, Rosenthal, Hall, DiMatteo, Rogers, & Archer, 1979).

M. Robin DiMatteo and her colleagues have conducted several studies in which physicians were administered a test of ability to decode the meanings of expressions conveyed in the face, body, and voice tone channels, and were also asked to pose or act out emotions using their voice or face and voice (reading standard-content passages to keep the verbal content ambiguous). In two studies, accuracy at judging emotions through the body channel was a significant predictor of how satisfied the physicians' patients were in their relationship with the physician (DiMatteo, 1979). In other words, physicians who could read body movement cues more accurately had more effective interpersonal relationships with their patients.

Other research has also implicated sensitivity to body cues in clinical psychologists' effectiveness (Rosenthal et al., 1979). The significance of reading the body in this research is no coincidence, since it is now established that some channels of nonverbal communication are less under conscious control than others, and are more likely to "leak" affect cues, even when a person is trying to cover up or contain them (Zuckerman & Driver, 1985). The body is one of these channels.

In a later study, physicians' ability to decode another leaky channel—the voice—was a significant predictor of their patients' compliance with scheduled appointments. Better decoders of emotions in the voice had patients who were more likely to show up as scheduled (DiMatteo, Hays, & Prince, 1986).

Ability to express emotions intentionally through nonverbal channels was also related to patient satisfaction (DiMatteo, 1979; DiMatteo et al., 1986). In particular, ability to express happy emotions seemed to be important. Physicians who were easily able to convey warmth, acceptance, and positive feelings toward patients seemed to be those whose patients returned a high level of regard. In this research, the physicians who were good expressors were also more dramatic, dominant, nonconforming, and playful on a battery of personality scales, and were rated as more likable in videotapes of their actual greetings with patients (Friedman, DiMatteo, & Taranta, 1980). Physicians who were good expressors also had more patients overall (DiMatteo et al., 1986).

THE EFFECTS OF MEDICAL TRAINING ON DOCTOR-PATIENT COMMUNICATION

As discussed earlier in this chapter, the process of becoming a doctor often starts with an early career decision and academic dedication designed to ensure a place in medical school. The educational process for physicians begins formally during the premed college years when eligibility for medical school is being determined. College undergraduates, determined to enter medical school, show signs and symptoms of what has been termed the premed syndrome—including "aggressive competitiveness, self-interested pursuit of grades, narrow minded overspecialization, high anxiety, and more than occasional incidents of academic dishonesty" (Fox, 1989, p. 98). These experiences are not inconsequential in molding and selecting the people who will ultimately become doctors, and they foreshadow the medical school experience.

Medical education is designed not only to teach biochemistry and physiology but to "transform an ordinary person into a doctor" (Bosk, 1979). How this transformation is accomplished during the process of medical education will have implications for the kind of doctor the student will become, and how that doctor will relate to his or her patients.

Critics of medical education have often argued that the emphasis on basic science is out of proportion with its relevance to clinical practice. Critical skills in communicating and relating to patients get short shrift in the medical curriculum. Indeed, in their early years of medical school, students do a better job of talking with their patients than fully trained doctors do. As students' medical education progresses, the science of medicine replaces its human dimension and students find it harder simply to talk with patients (Helfer, 1970). What were enjoyable talks with patients during the first years become awkward hypothesis-testing sessions later on. In other research, as training progressed students appeared to "miss the forest for the trees" and lose their grasp on the patient's total health picture in their single-minded focus on biomedical issues (Martin, Gilson, Bergner, Bobbitt, Pollard, Conn, & Cole, 1976).

The academic orientation of the student's medical school is instrumental in molding the way the student is likely to practice medicine and view his or her patients. One way to look at this issue is in terms of the tendency to use high technology or sophisticated tests. One such study found that the academic orientation of the medical school was related to test ordering (Epstein, Begg, & McNeil, 1984). The authors note that while it is possible that trainees with a predisposition to use technical services self-select into particular types of schools and training programs, it is also true that the environments of these schools develop clinical habits oriented toward high use of diagnostic tests.

Academically oriented schools produce physicians who rely heavily on tests because the role models in these schools are deeply involved in research and the use of technology for investigation, and this encourages the use of tests among young, impressionable students (Epstein et al., 1984). The biomedical emphasis in these schools is often at the expense of a more integrated appreciation of the patient's perspective and experience.

Internship and residency further reinforce biomedical and technological, as opposed to humanistic, considerations in regard to how young physicians view patients. The distancing of physicians from patients is accentuated in the hospital training experience in an alienating and punishing way. Despite the privileged backgrounds of most medical students, the hospital training experience is one of deprivation. The trainees are continually tested, both physically and emotionally, to prove their dedication to medicine with constant sleep deprivation and highly stressful work conditions (Butterfield, 1988).

A systematic, three-year observational study of the lives of interns and residents at a large university medical center was undertaken by sociologist Terry Mizrahi (1986). Mizrahi concludes that the most important lesson learned during the early months of training, and one that is reinforced throughout the trainee's career, is how to GROP (get rid of patients)—that is, discharge one's responsibility for patients as quickly as possible. "GROP became an art form within the house staff subculture, and those who were especially good at it were esteemed and called 'dispo kings' " (p. 166). Patients were seen as but one more obstacle to seeing their family or getting some sleep (Mizrahi, 1986). Mizrahi concludes that "the educational experience is structured to militate against the development of humanistic doctor-patient relationships. . . . [T]he novices [physicians in training] are systematically dehumanized, which only fosters the deterioration of the doctor-patient relationship rather than allowing it to develop as something positive" (p. 119).

All aspects of deprivation—psychological as well as physical—endured by interns and residents acted to extinguish any initial idealism and concern for patients the student may have had. Moreover, Mizrahi suggests that the frustrations experienced by the young doctors while in training were taken out on patients. In her words, it was a case of "one category of victims—albeit, temporary ones—victimizing a second weaker category" (Mizrahi, 1986, p. 166).

There were some exceptions to the GROP rule. Some patients were valued; patients who presented complex symptoms or a form of rare disease that could be used by the attending faculty and house staff for clinical material or teaching purposes were sought after. Further, it was noted that in addition to how interesting their case was, patients were classified on another continuum reflecting care burden and ranging from ideal to despised. The ideal patient was "middle class, intelligent without questioning the doctor's judgment, clean, deferential, helpful, cooperative, and so forth. The despised patient was one defined in the subculture as an abuser: a self-abuser, system abuser, house staff abuser or some combination" (Mizrahi, 1986, p. 167).

The extent of derision and bad feelings toward despised patients was reflected in a vocabulary of insults directed toward patients. GOMERS (get out of my emergency room), trainwrecks (patients with serious multiple medical problems), scumbags, dirtbags, crocks, garbage, junk, and SHPOS (subhuman pieces of shit) were terms repeatedly used to characterize patients, at times within earshot of the patient (Mizrahi, 1986). Any sympathy for patients was suppressed by an increasingly technical or procedural orientation toward patients, screening out any more subtle or subjective considerations. In this process, psychosocial and environmental factors were for the most part simply ignored, or under the best of circumstances deferred to others, most commonly social workers.

The experiences of young physicians described by Mizrahi have been recognized by a growing public awareness of the negative impact of training-related stress on both young physicians and their patients. Issues of medical malpractice have been raised by the lay press, the concern being that overworked and sleep-deprived residents may be prone to make serious and sometimes deadly mistakes (Asch & Parker, 1988). And, for the first time, prestigious residency programs in internal medicine have failed to find sufficient numbers of applicants to fill their residency slots, at least in some part due to dissatisfaction with the residency training process (Colford & McPhee, 1989). In fact, many medical educators now believe that the stresses of residency training have reached crisis proportions, and they are calling for a restructuring of the training experience. Commentators in this area feel that change is imminent as it becomes increasingly clear to society that the current process of training physicians is dangerous to both the trainees and their patients (Colford & McPhee, 1989).

There is some hope, however, that the damaging effects of training diminish over time. Several of the physicians observed throughout their training in the Mizrahi study were interviewed five and six years later (Mizrahi, 1986). The doctors in the follow-up were found to have softened their views of patients to some extent. In particular, those physicians who went into private practice, as opposed to academic medicine, had redefined their notion of optimal health care by decreasing the importance of technical and academic expertise and increasing the importance of considering the whole patient (Mizrahi, 1986).

REFERENCES

Asch, D., & Parker, R. (1988). The Libby Zion case. *New England Journal of Medicine, 318*, 771–774.

Bosk, C. L. (1979). *Forgive and remember: Managing medical failure.* Chicago: University of Chicago Press.

Butterfield, P. (1988). The stress of residency: A review of the literature. *Archives of Internal Medicine, 148*, 1428–1435.

Coe, R. M. (1970). *Sociology of medicine.* New York: McGraw Hill.

Colford, J. M., & McPhee, S. J. (1989). The ravelled sleeve of care: Managing the stresses of residency training. *Journal of the American Medical Association, 261*, 889–893.

Cypress, B. K. (1980). Characteristics of visits to female and male physicians. Vital and Health Statistics, series 13, no. 49. Hyattsville, Md.: U.S. Department of Health and Human Services.

DiMatteo, M. R. (1979). Nonverbal skill and the physician-patient relationship. In Rosenthal, R. (Ed.), *Skill in nonverbal communication: Individual differences.* Cambridge, Mass.: Oelgeschlager, Gunn & Hain.

DiMatteo, M. R., Hays, R. D., & Prince, L. M. (1986). Relationship of physicians' nonverbal communication skill to patient satisfaction, appointment noncompliance, and physician workload. *Health Psychology, 5*, 581–594.

Eisenberg, J. (1986). *Doctors' decisions and the cost of medical care.* Ann Arbor, Mich.: Health Administration Press.

Epstein, A. M., Begg, C. B., & McNeil, B. J. (1984). The effects of physicians' training and personality on test ordering for ambulatory patients. *American Journal of Public Health, 74*, 1271–1273.

Fox, R. (1989). *Essays in medical sociology: Journeys into the field.* New Brunswick, N.J.: Transaction Books.

Freidson, E. (1970a). *Profession of medicine: A study of the sociology of applied knowledge.* New York: Dodd Mead.

Freidson, E. (1975). *Doctoring together: A study of professional social control.* New York: Elsevier.

Friedman, H. S., DiMatteo, M. R., & Taranta, A. (1980). A study of the relationship between individual differences in nonverbal expressiveness and factors of personality and social interaction. *Journal of Research in Personality, 14*, 351–364.

Hall, J. A. (1984). *Nonverbal sex differences: Communication accuracy and expressive style.* Baltimore: Johns Hopkins University Press.

Hall, J. A., Epstein, A. M., DeCiantis, M. L., & McNeil, B. J. (1993). Physicians' liking for their patients: More evidence for the role of affect in medical care. *Health Psychology*, forthcoming.

Hall, O. (1948). The stages of a medical career. *American Journal of Sociology, 53*, 327–336.

Haug, M., & Lavin, B. (1983). *Consumerism in medicine: Challenging physician authority.* Beverly Hills, Calif.: Sage Publications.

Helfer, R. E. (1970). An objective comparison of the pediatric interviewing skills of freshman and senior medical students. *Pediatrics*, *45*, 623–627.

Hollingshead, A. B., & Redlich, F. C. (1958). *Social class and mental illness*. New York: John Wiley & Sons.

Jonas, H. S., & Etzel, S. (1988). Undergraduate medical education. *Journal of the American Medical Association*, *260*, 1063–1071.

Kurtz, R. A., & Chalfant, H. P. (1991). *The sociology of medicine and illness*. 2nd ed. Boston: Allyn & Bacon.

Light, D. (1975). The sociological calendar: An analytic tool for fieldwork applied to medical and psychiatric training. *American Journal of Sociology*, *80*, 1145–1164.

Linn, L. S., & Lewis, C. E. (1979). Attitudes toward self-care among practicing physicians. *Medical Care*, *17*, 183–190.

Martin, D. P., Gilson, B. S., Bergner, M., Bobbitt, R. A., Pollard, W. E., Conn, J. R., & Cole, W. A. (1976). The Sickness Impact Profile: Potential use of a health status instrument for physician training. *Journal of Medical Education*, *51*, 942–947.

Mechanic, D. (1974). *Politics, medicine, and social science*. New York: John Wiley & Sons.

Mechanic, D. (1978). *Medical sociology*, 2nd ed. New York: The Free Press.

Mizrahi, T. (1986). *Getting rid of patients: Contradictions in the socialization of physicians*. New Brunswick, N.J.: Rutgers University Press.

Ornstein, S. M., Markert, G. P., Johnson, A. H., Rust, P. F., & Afrin, L. B. (1988). The effect of physician personality on laboratory test ordering for hypertensive patients. *Medical Care*, *26*, 536–543.

Rogoff, N. (1957). The decision to study medicine. In Merton, R. K., Reader, G. G., & Kendall, P. L. (Eds.), *The student-physician*. Cambridge, Mass.: Harvard University Press.

Rosengren, W. R. (1980). *Sociology of medicine: Diversity, conflict and change*. New York: Harper & Row.

Rosenthal, R., Hall, J. A., DiMatteo, M. R., Rogers, P. L., & Archer, D. (1979). *Sensitivity to nonverbal communication: The PONS test*. Baltimore: Johns Hopkins University Press.

Roter, D., Lipkin, M., Jr., & Korsgaard, A. (1991). Sex differences in patients' and physicians' communication during primary care medical visits. *Medical Care*, *29*, 1083–1093.

Scully, D. (1980). *Men who control women's health: The miseducation of obstetrician-gynecologists*. Boston: Houghton Mifflin.

Tudor, C. (1988). Career plans and debt levels of graduating U.S. medical students, 1981–1986. *Journal of Medical Education*, *63*, 271–275.

Waitzkin, H. (1985). Information giving in medical care. *Journal of Health and Social Behavior*, *26*, 81–101.

Waitzkin, H., & Waterman, B. (1974). *The exploitation of illness in capitalist society*. New York: Bobbs-Merrill.

Wasserman, R. C., Inui, T. S., Barriatua, R. D., Carter, W. B., & Lippincott, P. (1984). Pediatric clinicians' support for parents makes a difference: An outcome-based analysis of clinician-parent interaction. *Pediatrics*, *74*, 1047–1053.
Zuckerman, M., & Driver, R. E. (1985). Telling lies: Verbal and nonverbal correlates of deception. In Siegman, A. W., & Feldstein, S. (Eds.), *Multichannel integrations of nonverbal behavior*. Hillsdale, N.J.: Erlbaum.

Part II

What Usually Happens in Medical Visits

5

Patterns of Talk in the Medical Visit

By most estimates, the average primary care medical visit in the United States lasts less than twenty minutes—about fourteen minutes for family practice and nineteen minutes for internal medicine (Nelson & McLemore, 1988). Although there is a good deal of variation, with some visits as short as thirty seconds and others as long as an hour or more, most of the complicated business of healing is accomplished in relatively short, sporadic encounters. In this chapter the medical encounter will be described, including what a doctor is likely to say and what a patient is likely to say back. For the most part, the description will reflect visits to doctors' offices, although for a point of reference it will relate what we know about patients' talk with doctors in the hospital. The charts and figures presented in this chapter are based on actual observation of thousands of routine medical encounters.

Direct observation of medical visits has not had a very long tradition. Despite intense interest in the therapeutic encounter dating back to the days of Hippocrates, it has only been since the late 1960s, with advances in recording technology, that the medical encounter has been systematically observed. Perhaps because of the physical exposure of the exam there is an element of privacy to the medical visit that has discouraged the researcher's intrusion. But physical exposure is only one aspect of the visit that is considered private; discovery of illness, and the fears and vulnerabilities that may accompany it, are also intensely private. Legal structures and professional ethics have surrounded the visit to ensure that these discussions can be open and free from fear. Confidentiality is jealously guarded. In an emotional, physical, as well as legal sense, the talk between doctor and patient and its documentation in a patient's chart are treated as privileged communication.

In light of the high regard and protective structures surrounding the privacy of the medical visit, it is surprising that physicians and patients are willing to have their visits studied at all. However, they usually are. In the largest published study of routine medical interaction (Byrne & Long, 1976), based on more than 1,200 patients and 160 physicians in private practice, it was reported that fewer than 5% of the patients who were asked refused to participate. In our own studies, we find a 10% to 20% refusal rate—about what you would expect in any research project.

What these patients and physicians are agreeing to, with assurances that their names or any other identifiers will not be used, is most often tape recording of their entire medical visit. Occasionally, a nonparticipant observer, a researcher who observes or takes notes during the medical visit but who does not participate in any way, is present. Virtually all studies provide participants with the option to withdraw from the study, turn the tape recorder off for any period of time, or ask the observer to leave; however, this is rarely done.

One may wonder whether the presence of an observer or recorder inhibits or changes what goes on between the patient and doctor. An infringement of the privacy of the medical visit, an invasion of its privileged communication, could somehow violate its very nature. This does not appear to happen. Both patients and doctors report forgetting about the tape recorder soon after the visit begins, and few have indicated that the recorders changed their visits in any way. Moreover, diversity of both patient and physician behavior observed through these tapes reflects the frank and open manner in which they were made. Byrne and Long (1976) note that the many incidents of physician failure with patients included in their study make the likelihood of censored behavior or especially selected visits on the part of the physicians unlikely. In our own studies, the great range of physician behavior in the audiotapes we have studied also points to little conscious manipulation of behavior in any particular way.

Tape recordings are used to provide researchers with more than just a verbatim record of what is said during the medical visit; they are more revealing than one might at first think. For one thing, some of the nonverbal communication of the encounter can be captured. Coders are able to rate the emotional tone of each speaker during the visit based on an overall impression created by both what is said and how it is said; that is, the specific content of the dialogue and also the voice quality of the participants can be studied. Of course, when videotapes are made, an even richer record is available.

In some studies of tape recordings, we have gone further in assessment of emotional tone and have analyzed patient and physician voice quality independent of the specific dialogue (Hall, Roter, & Rand, 1981; Hall, Roter, & Katz, 1988). To do this, we made the doctor's and patient's words unintelligible by passing the audiotape through an electronic filter that removed specified frequency bands from the speech. The resulting filtered speech is muffled so that words cannot be understood, but expressive features such as pitch, speed, and rhythm remain. Segments of this filtered tape are then played for judges, who rate what they hear for the expressed intensity of a variety of emotions, such as anger, anxiety, dominance, interest, and friendliness.

While the assessment of nonverbal aspects of communication may seem complicated, analysis of verbal communication can seem overwhelming. The diversity of patient and physician behavior suggests a multitude of communication variables to study. In our review of sixty-one published studies in the field prior to 1987 (Hall, Roter, & Katz, 1988; Roter, Hall, & Katz, 1988), we found 247 unique communication variables abstracted from observations of patient and physician interaction. Few of the variables, at least in the form in which they were reported, were common to more than one or two studies. However, virtually all of the variables fit within five mutually exclusive categories: information giving, question asking or information seeking, social conversation, positive talk, and negative talk. An additional category, partnership building, applied to physician interaction only. Specific items falling within these categories are given in Tables 5.1 and 5.2 to give readers a feel for the different ways in which these kinds of communication were defined.

How this table translates to a portrait of the medical encounter in terms of actual frequencies of each category is displayed in Table 5.3. Reviewing physician talk (Table 5.3), we found that what they do most is give information. This includes all forms of information giving, as reflected by the subcategories listed on Table 5.1. For some physicians this consists of a mere recital of facts ("Your blood pressure is high today, 180/95."). Others offer counseling ("It is very important that you take all the medication I am prescribing. You have to get your blood pressure under control, and this medication will do it, but only if you take it as you are supposed to."); or directions and instructions ("Put your clothes back on and sit down. Now, take these pills twice a day for a week and drink plenty of water."). Each of these approaches has a different intent—to inform, to persuade, or to control, respectively.

From our own work it appears that the giving of facts makes up about half of the information-giving category, and both counseling and directing patient behavior contribute in equal parts to the remainder. The next chapter will be

Table 5.1
Specific Variables Included in Physician Categories

1. *Information giving:* Gives information, gives opinion, gives suggestion, gives instruction, percentage of communication that is educational, gives explanation, gives information and orientation, explains, discusses problem resolution, offers descriptive communication, answers patient questions, discloses, gives information on: patient condition, nature of illness, cause, symptoms, diagnosis, current health treatment, nonmedical treatment, medical treatment, self-care, physical activity, diet, health promotion, lifestyle.

2. *Information seeking:* Asks for information, asks for instructions, takes medical history, asks about compliance (open-ended and closed-ended questions), percentage of communication that is questions, asks for patient questions, seeks patient ideas.

3. *Social conversation:* Greetings, nonmedical statements (social conversation, greetings), personal remarks, social remarks, casual conversation, discusses social/family matters.

4. *Positive talk:* Agrees, shows approval, laughs, shows solidarity, gives reassurance, offers support, facilitates, encourages, shows empathy, calms patient, percentage of communication with positive content.

5. *Negative talk:* Disagrees, confronts, shows antagonism, shows tension.

6. *Partnership building:* Asks for patient opinion, asks for understanding, asks for suggestions, requests questions, seeks patient ideas, makes interpretations, reflects patients' statements, facilitates patient response, makes acknowledgment.

devoted to a deeper exploration of information and its importance in the medical visit.

Physicians' asking of questions also accounts for a good proportion of the visit; this is usually done during history taking and mostly consists of closed-ended questions. Closed-ended questions are those questions for which a one-word answer, usually yes or no, is expected (e.g., "Are your leg symptoms worse after standing for several minutes?"). In contrast, questions that allow patients some discretion in the direction they may take in answering are open-ended questions (e.g., "Tell me about your leg pain. What seems to be the problem?").

Considering the complexities of diagnostic reasoning, patients are hard-pressed to know what it is about their symptoms or medical history that the physician might consider relevant to their current problem. Physician questions provide the cues that patients take in deciding what it is they should tell the doctor.

Table 5.2
Specific Variables Included in Patient Categories

1. *Information giving:* Presents symptoms, answers questions, responds to instructions, offers problem-related experience, gives suggestions, opinion, orientation, information.

2. *Information seeking:* Asks for orientation, opinion, instruction, suggestions, asks questions (general), asks questions about medication, treatment, lifestyle, prevention, self-care.

3. *Social conversation:* Social exchange, social remarks, introductory phrases, nonmedical social conversation, family/social conversation (not psychosocial exchanges).

4. *Positive talk:* Laughter, friendliness, display of solidarity, tension release, agreement, show of approval.

5. *Negative talk:* Shows antagonism, disagrees, shows tension.

Closed-ended questions limit responses to a narrow field set by the physician; the patient knows that an appropriate response is one or two words and does not normally elaborate any further. In contrast, open-ended questions suggest to the patient that elaboration is appropriate and that the field of inquiry is wide enough to include patient thoughts about what might be relevant. These two types of questions have very different implications for control of the medical visit; closed-ended questions imply high physician control of the interaction while open-ended questions are much less controlling.

Closed-ended questions are often posed as a method of testing a hypothesis; it is assumed that if a physician is on the right track, and has a fair sense of what the patient's problem is, these questions are efficient prompts to the patient to give the physician the information needed. Open-ended questions, on the other hand, are often suggested when there is hypothesis uncertainty. If the physician does not have a clear idea of the underlying problem, open-ended questions can help orient him or her and provide a starting point. In routine practice, closed-ended questions far outnumber open-ended questions, by a factor of two or three, and they are thought to be less time-consuming and more efficient at getting the physician the information needed to make a diagnosis.

Our own work sheds some light on these questions (Roter & Hall, 1987). Contrary to the widespread practice favoring closed-ended questions, we found that open-ended questions prompted the revelation of substantially more relevant information by patients than closed-ended questions.

Positive talk makes up a smaller share of physician talk, only half as much as questions, and serves two functions. One is obvious. Approval (e.g., "Your blood pressure is great! You've been doing a good job on your diet and taking your pills."), as well as shared laughter, encouragement, and empathy all increase a positive bond between doctor and patient. The second purpose of statements in this category is to signal that one is attentive and eager for the speaker to continue. Often included are communications more aptly described as noises than words: hm, huh, aha, and ahh serve this purpose. A study focusing on the first ninety seconds of the visit found that the more a physician used these noises, the more likely he or she was to uncover fully the patient's major concerns and reason for the visit (Beckman & Frankel, 1984). Patients readily defer to the physician and are easily diverted from giving their thoughts. Attentive noises encourage elaboration, so that a patient's full agenda for the visit can be revealed.

Partnership building represents the physician's attempts to engage the patient more fully in the medical dialogue. These may be considered, in some respect, as attempts to activate the patient, perhaps directed at particularly passive or noncommunicative patients.

Social, nonmedical conversation makes up some 5% of interaction. It includes greetings, casual remarks, and niceties ("Hello Mr. Waller, nice to see you. That was some baseball game last night."). This talk is important as a social amenity—it is usually positive, and we are accustomed to greetings and a certain amount of chit-chat in most encounters, at least initially, to put people at ease.

Finally, negative talk, as is obvious from Table 5.3, is quite rare from physicians. This includes disagreements, confrontations, and antagonisms ("You've gained weight since your last visit and I am disappointed in you. You're not really trying at all."). It is probably a good guess that while negative talk is not often made explicit by physicians, the intent is still expressed and negative emotional messages are conveyed. Professional etiquette and training discourage unpleasantness and the high emotions that may arise from direct criticisms and contradictions. Our research implies that physicians find other ways to express displeasure. Reprimands may be expressed as forceful counseling or imperatives on the need to follow recommendations better. In the case of an unsuccessful dieter, for instance, this could mean exhortation for the patient to do better on the diet and follow a prescribed regimen. The physician may also express displeasure in an angry, anxious, or dominant tone of voice, and by cutting patients off in various ways.

Although there are many ways in which physicians and patients may engage in reciprocal behavior, analyses of voice quality and other nonverbal behaviors reveal an especially subtle, and possibly unconscious, demonstration of reciprocity. Using electronically filtered excerpts of speech (excerpts in which the words are made to be unintelligible but the affective qualities

Table 5.3
Profile of Physician Interaction

Variable	# Studies	Range	Mean	Median	Weighted Mean	S.D.
Information Giving	12	4-60%	35.3%	38.5%	24.8%	16.90
Information Seeking	12	6-40%	22.6%	22.5%	20.1%	9.61
Social Conversation	6	5-10%	6.0%	5.0%	5.4%	1.83
Positive Talk	10	1-31%	15.0%	14.5%	11.9%	9.27
Negative Talk	3	.5-2.5%	1.3%	1.0%	2.3%	0.94
Partnership Building	7	3-25%	10.6%	10.0%	8.8%	6.52

of the voice remain), Hall, Roter, and Rand (1981) found in fifty outpatient visits strong evidence that the voice tone of doctors and patients was correlated. Independent judges' ratings of emotional qualities in separate tapes of doctors' and patients' speech showed that when the doctor sounded angry, anxious, or contented, so did the patient (and vice versa). Thus, they mirrored each other's vocal affect. This prompts one to ask whether one participant sets the tone and the other follows, or whether they each reflect back the other's affect in a spiraling fashion? If so, we can imagine both positive and negative spirals. Of course the negative spiral is the most dangerous, and all the more so because individuals rarely appreciate that their own behavior has produced the other's response. Thus, the grumpy patient whose doctor responds grumpily will likely attribute the doctor's behavior to negative personal qualities or attitudes, without realizing that the doctor was simply responding in kind to the patient's own behavior. Perhaps it is no surprise that the doctor's and patient's satisfaction with the visit are positively correlated—when one is happy with the visit, so is the other.

A study of ours on one hundred outpatient visits, mentioned in Chapter 3, also finds evidence for communication reciprocity. Significant reciprocity, or matching, between physician and patient was found for the use of tag

Table 5.4
Profile of Patient Interaction

Variable	# Studies	Range	Mean	Median	Weighted Mean	S.D.
Information Giving	9	28-67%	46.9%	54.0%	43.5%	14.50
Question Asking	9	2.6-14.5%	7.0%	6.0%	6.1%	3.53
Social Conversation	5	4-42%	13.4%	7.0%	5.7%	14.40
Positive Talk	4	11-23%	18.7%	20.5%	20.11%	4.92
Negative Talk	3	5-13%	8.3%	7.0%	9.5%	3.40

questions (e.g., "They really make you wait a long time, *don't they?*"); social chit-chat; amount of psychosocial information revealed; and filtered speech ratings of friendliness, anxiety, and boredom. Other behaviors showed reciprocity for one sex but not the other, or occasionally negative reciprocity. For female patients, the number of successful interruptions was positively correlated between doctor and patient, but for male patients this relation was opposite in nature: the more the doctor interrupted, the less the patient did, and vice versa.

Physicians almost always talk more than patients during medical visits. This is something of a surprise to physicians—they generally overestimate the amount of patient talk and underestimate their own talk. The relative amount of patient and physician contribution to the medical dialogue averages around 40% by patients and 60% by physicians.

As reflected in Table 5.4, patient interaction falls within several primary categories. It should not be surprising to find that more than half of patient talk is information giving, and much of this is patient response to physician questions. What is surprising, however, is how little time during the visit, some 6%, is taken in patients asking questions. This is particularly troubling since many studies have demonstrated that patients often have questions they would like to ask but simply do not. Such reticence may reflect a reluctance to appear foolish or inappropriate; or it may be that physicians, in myriad ways, signal that the time is not right to ask questions. The right time, however, is never quite there. Whatever the reason, questions from patients are relatively rare.

Negative talk reported in the studies we reviewed was seven times as great for patients as for physicians. It is notable how much more frequent direct contradiction or criticism of the physician is by the patient than vice versa. Patients may be more direct in this regard than their physicians since they have fewer communication options; they cannot easily express their disagreements through lecture, counseling, or imperatives. However, patients engage in more positive as well as negative talk. The expression of these emotionally laden statements generally marks greater interpersonal engagement. The patient is likely to have a far greater emotional investment in the proceedings than the physician, and this is expressed in both positive and negative terms.

The less than twenty minutes we refer to as the length of an average visit reflects more than actual time spent talking. It often includes fairly lengthy periods of silence, in which the physician is attending to something other than the patient. Interruptions during a visit by a telephone call from another patient or doctor are not uncommon; there are also buzzes from the receptionist and a nurse's head appearing in the door asking for clarification of a schedule or order. In our large study of routine medical visits we found that 30% of the visits had at least one interruption.

Interruptions of another kind are also common. Doctors often begin and end a visit with the medical record rather than the patient. The first few minutes of a visit are often devoted to a review of prior notes or consultant letters, and the conclusion of the visit is often taken with several minutes of note taking, prescription writing, and the completion of test orders.

Half the time allotted to a patient's visit can easily be taken with activities in which the patient's presence is not needed and is, in fact, ignored.

To make matters worse, an English study of appointment scheduling found that the time of day at which a visit is scheduled affects the amount of time the doctor spends with the patient (Byrne & Long, 1976). Patients seen early in the day had visits from 10% to 40% longer than the average, while patients seen during the late afternoon had visits from 25% to 50% shorter than the average. It was clear that early in the day the doctors were more relaxed and took more time with their patients, but by midafternoon the pressure to complete their patient schedule led to shorter visits. The doctors in the study were surprised at the findings; they were completely unaware of these differences.

Having presented some bare statistics about talk during the medical visit, one might ask how relevant it is to any given medical encounter between a particular doctor and an individual patient.

Several perspectives on the doctor-patient relationship provide somewhat different expectations as to how a given visit is likely to proceed. The first, a sociological perspective, predicts that both patients and physicians operate closely within a framework of social roles, which "script" the way in which the visit will be acted out. Far from being spontaneous, the visit really reflects a well-rehearsed exchange in which certain things are supposed to happen. The implication of this view is that most patients act pretty much the same and are treated more or less the same as other patients.

Alternatively, one might suggest that it is the unique qualities of the patient and his or her particular problem that make each case different from any other, and that consequently each encounter with the doctor is finely tailored to account for these clinical differences. Akin to the clinical differences view is a perspective that it is the patient's personality that affects treatment; likable patients may be talked to differently than difficult or problem patients. This suggests that physicians are sensitive to individual patient differences and that communication reflects these differences.

Rather than individual differences, sociologists claim that it is the host of demographic and social characteristics, such as the patient's age, sex, race, social class, and income, that drive the way in which the visit will go. These class differences have implications for how the patient will act, and how the provider will react to particular groups of patients. Since the majority of physicians are white, male, and middle class, they would be expected to act (or react) in a predictable manner to different classes of patients.

Each of the views has in common the assumption that patients, in one way or another—by virtue of their conception of the patient role, or by their clinical problem, or personality, or class membership—dictate the way in which they are likely to be treated. These assumptions reflect a widespread belief that physicians vary their mode of communication to accommodate patient differences.

A different perspective, however, may be gained by considering the opposite view—that is, that individual physicians are quite consistent in their communication style and relate to all of their patients in a similar manner, largely ignoring individual patient differences. Further, not only are physicians committed to a rather enduring style of communication, there is a great deal of variation among doctors.

A useful insight into this controversy was provided by four patients in the same practice who were seen by several doctors of that practice participating in an audiotape study of communication (Byrne & Long, 1976). On one of these visits, the patients saw doctors other than their usual physicians because of scheduling constraints. In every case the behavior of the patient was markedly different from that exhibited with his or her regular physician. Two of the patients were much more inhibited and less communicative, while the other two were much more communicative. The two patients who became less communicative were seen by a doctor who had an interviewing style in which he exercised much more control over his patients than other doctors in the practice. When the patients of the controlling doctor saw other doctors with less controlling styles, they engaged in a much greater and detailed exchange than they had with their usual doctor. The conclusion of these researchers was that patients appeared to be accommodating to the comparatively inflexible styles of their doctors.

Style in communication, as in dress or art or cooking, reflects an underlying consistency with which a repertoire of behaviors is expressed. We have found in our own work, as have several other researchers exploring this issue, that physician style can be characterized as doctor-centered or patient-centered. Doctor-centered communication is intended to meet the physician's agenda: the gathering of sufficient information to test hypotheses in order to make a diagnosis and recommend treatment, and the need to have the visit proceed quickly and efficiently. Giving of directions and asking questions (which is largely dominated by closed-ended questions) are communication strategies that may be considered physician-centered. Directions, for the most part, are given to keep the visit moving by managing the patient during the physical exam. For example, this category includes statements such as "open your mouth" and "get on the table." The asking of questions also reflects physician dominance in directing the interview and limiting patient comments to those areas specified by the doctor.

The need to control the visit is summed up in the comments of a physician who participated in the English study of communication: "The doctor's primary task is to manage his time. If he allows patients to rabbit on about their conditions then the doctor will lose control of time and will spend all his time sitting in a surgery listening to irrelevant rubbish. Effective doctoring is characterized by a 'quick clean job'" (Byrne & Long, 1976, p. 93).

Although doctor-centered communication may be effective in maintaining the doctor's control of the visit, this type of communication is less successful in addressing patient needs. Coupled with the desire for a cure or relief of pain, patients need to make sense of a frightening and new experience associated with illness (Stoeckle & Barsky, 1981). Information giving, counseling, open-ended questions, interpretation and paraphrase to assure comprehension, request for opinion, confirming comprehension, reassurance, and statements of concern, agreement, and approval are all examples of physicians' communication behaviors that are patient-centered and have relevance for patient goals.

Patient-centered exchanges maximize a collaboration between both doctors and patients, while, one might suggest, doctor-centered exchanges maximize the physician's input and minimize the value of patient input. An example of this difference is illustrated in the following brief prescribing exchanges between physicians and patients with the same basic diagnosis of upper respiratory tract infection:

You have an upper respiratory tract infection. More likely than not it will clear itself up in three or four days. I can give a prescription that may well clear it faster. What do you think? (patient-centered)

Take this to the drug store and come back in a week if it is not better. (physician-centered)

Social, nonmedical conversation cannot be clearly viewed in terms of either patient-centered or doctor-centered talk. This category presents some difficulty. On the one hand, social talk is important as a social amenity—it is usually positive and it may help put people at ease. Too much nonmedical talk, however, may be perceived as reflecting a casual attitude or lack of concentration. There is likely to be a threshold level below which this kind of talk may be regarded as patient-centered, fulfilling a need for rapport and ease, but beyond which it is less functional for the patient.

As an illustration, consider the experience of Mrs. W. (a real patient). She had a particularly unsatisfying visit with one of her obstetrical doctors when she was pregnant, and spent some time trying to figure out what went wrong. Much of the visit time was taken by the physician telling her about his daughter. At first, Mrs. W. felt pleased that the physician was sharing an aspect of his personal life, but after several minutes the discussion began to feel inappropriate. She felt powerless to stop or redirect the physician's monologue and simply nodded throughout. Afterward, she was furious because her time had been taken with the doctor's need to talk about his daughter while Mrs. W. wanted to talk about her baby!

In our own study of physician style among forty-three male doctors in Pennsylvania (Hall, Roter, & Katz, 1987), we found a strong trade-off effect between physician-centered and patient-centered communication, as well as between nonmedical, social talk and patient-centered communication. We found that the more patient-centered the doctor (the more informative and likely to give counseling), the less time the doctor spent in social talk, asking questions, and directing the visit. If this pattern held true in Mrs. W.'s visit, then it was likely that the doctor not only spent a good deal of the visit in social talk but compensated by spending less time in giving her information and counseling relevant to the pregnancy.

We also found relationships between nonverbal communication and patient-centered and physician-centered styles in this study. We found that physicians who presented more medical information and less social talk to their patients had a voice quality that sounded more interested and more anxious than physicians who presented less medical information and more social talk. Physicians who are more oriented toward medical information delivery and who neglect social conversation may compensate for this neglect by the more alert, interested quality of their voices. Conversely, it appears that physicians who gave less information spent more time in pleasantries but had voices that were perceived as bored and calm. Based on this study, and others (Hall, Roter, & Rand, 1981), we believe that within the context of the medical encounter, anxiety in the physician's voice is perceived positively as reflecting anxious regard. Particularly when coupled with greater signs of interest, we believe that informative physicians create an impression of sincerity, dedication, and competence. The possible negative impact of the combination of boredom and calm for the less informative doctors may not be offset by the content of positive social conversation.

In our study, we were able to make use of data collected by an earlier team of researchers (Wang, Terry, Flynn, Williamson, Green, & Faden, 1979), which indicated how well the physicians performed on 150 behaviors. These, based on transcripts of the medical visit, included ordering appropriate tests, prescribing the correct medications, taking a good history, and offering appropriate information. We found that physician-centered communications (i.e., giving directions, asking questions) and social conversation were all negatively associated with these clinical proficiency scores. On the other hand, patient-centered communications (i.e., giving information and coun-seling) were positively associated with proficiency.

The physicians who had a patient-centered style of communication left a more positive impression on patients. Moreover these physicians were, in fact, more competent than other doctors (Hall & Roter, 1988). They scored higher on the pencil-and-paper tests that reflect "book learning," as well as actually engaging in more of the behaviors during the medical visit deemed appropriate by the expert panel of physicians.

We don't infer from these findings in isolation that physicians should abandon social conversation, or that a physician who is socially chatty is necessarily incompetent. There may be an important minimum threshold for social niceties that creates a friendly atmosphere that is appreciated by both doctor and patient. However, too much social conversation may take visit time away from information giving and counseling on the part of the physician and make it more difficult for the patient to provide the important psychosocial and biomedical information that provides insight into his or her illness experience and medical condition. Furthermore, there may be a basis for suspecting that a physician who makes this trade-off and spends too much time in social chit-chat may be less competent than other physicians.

REFERENCES

Beckman, H. B., & Frankel, R. M. (1984). The effect of physician behavior on the collection of data. *Annals of Internal Medicine*, *101*, 692–696.

Byrne, P. S., & Long, B.E.L. (1976). *Doctors talking to patients*. London: Her Majesty's Stationery Office.

Hall, J. A., & Roter, D. L. (1988). Physicians' knowledge and self-reported compliance promotion as predictors of performance with simulated lung disease patients. *Evaluation and the Health Professions*, *11*, 306–317.

Hall, J. A., Roter, D. L., & Katz, N. R. (1988). Meta-analysis of correlates of provider behavior in medical encounters. *Medical Care*, *26*, 657–675.

Hall, J. A., Roter, D. L., & Rand, C. S. (1981). Communication of affect between patient and physician. *Journal of Health and Social Behavior*, *22*, 18–30.

Nelson, C., & McLemore, T. (1988). National Center for Health Statistics. The National Ambulatory Medical Care Survey: U.S. 1975–81, and 1985 trends. Vital and Health Statistics, series 13, no. 93, DHHS pub. no. (PHS) 88–1754. Washington, D.C.: U.S. Government Printing Office.

Roter, D. L., & Hall, J. A. (1987). Physicians' interviewing styles and medical information obtained from patients. *Journal of General Internal Medicine*, *2*, 325–329.

Roter, D. L., Hall, J. A., & Katz, N. R. (1988). Physician-patient communication: A descriptive summary of the literature. *Patient Education and Counseling*, *12*, 99–119.

Stoeckle, J. D., & Barsky, A. (1981). Attributions: Uses of social science knowledge in doctoring in primary care. In Eisenberg, L., & Kleinman, A. (Eds.), *The relevance of social science for medicine*. Boston: D. Reidel.

Wang, V., Terry, P., Flynn, B., Williamson, J., Green, L., & Faden, R. (1979). Evaluation of continuing medical education for chronic obstructive pulmonary diseases. *Journal of Medical Education*, *54*, 803–811.

6

Giving and Withholding Information: The Special Case of Informative Talk in the Medical Visit

Part of the mystique of medicine is that it is written and often communicated in a foreign code. To make matters worse, the code has two forms: the scientific, anatomical, and technologically correct usage of terms to describe body parts, body processes, medical procedures, and medical treatments; and an even more impenetrable shorthand for these things, used in hospitals and medical records. There is some evidence that physicians themselves have trouble understanding this code (Christy, 1979).

"Medicalese" persists despite its difficulties, and if a patient feels alarmed and confused after leaving the doctor's office, it is not unusual. It is a good guess that a doctor will use at least one unfamiliar medical term in any given visit. Barbara Korsch and her colleagues (Korsch, Gozzi, & Francis, 1968) found that the pediatrician's use of difficult technical language and medical shorthand was a barrier to communication in more than half of the eight hundred pediatric visits that were studied. Mothers were often confused and unsure of terms used by the doctor to describe what was wrong with their children and what the doctor was going to do about it. Although one mother asked the doctor to repeat what he said "in English," this kind of confrontation appeared infrequent; for the most part, mothers did not ask for clarification of unfamiliar terms.

Other researchers similarly report that patients are confused, but are reluctant to ask for clarification. For instance, after observing over 150 medical visits, Svarstad (1974) found that both patients and doctors engaged in a kind of communication conspiracy. Physicians generally spoke as though their patients understood them, and patients acted as though that was indeed the case, even though this was far from the truth. In only 15% of the visits in which an unfamiliar term was used did patients actually tell the doctor that they did not recognize or understand the term. Most often, the patient simply remained silent. Fear of appearing ignorant is the reason most often given by patients for failing to ask doctors what they mean when technical terms are used. In addition to their confusion, patients often find themselves in something of a bind: it is flattering to have the physician assume they understand the fancy language, and this in itself makes it hard to admit otherwise (Korsch et al., 1968).

Our research on one hundred medical visits at a major teaching hospital (see Chapter 3) confirms that many words are used without explanation. Here is a sample of unexplained terms used by the fifty physicians in that study:

temporomandibular joint
electrolytes
stool guiac
sigmoidoscopy
circadian rhythm
creatinine
hypothyroid
infiltrate
aneurysm
dysrhythmic
tricyclics

In some cases, the patient may have known the words because of prior interactions with the physician. Nevertheless, since in this dataset the great majority of medical and technical words were given without explanation, we are skeptical that patients entered their visits that well informed.

In this study, the more junior physicians, including medical residents, were more likely to use jargon than were the more senior ones. Yet junior physicians were also more likely to give explanations, while not being significantly more likely to receive requests for explanations. Thus, less experienced physicians may both show off their knowledge of esoteric terms and feel the need to tell the patient what they mean. An alternative interpretation of the seniority effect may be that younger physicians feel more on a par with patients and feel less of a need to talk down (by simplifying their language) than do higher-ranking physicians.

There is evidence that doctors are not unaware of the problems patients have in following their technical explanations. Several studies indicate that, if anything, physicians generally underestimate what patients understand

(McKinlay, 1975). In a particularly telling study, physicians were asked to identify terms they thought their patients would have difficulty understanding. The researchers found that many of these terms were actually used during the medical visit by these very doctors, in disregard of the reservations they had expressed. The physicians used these terms even though they did not expect their patients to understand them (McKinlay, 1975).

Why would doctors intentionally use terms they knew their patients did not understand? Medical sociologists offer two somewhat contradictory perceptions of the patient to explain physicians' disinclination to communicate information. The first is a view of the patient as incompetent to comprehend or cope emotionally with medical information. This view assumes that, lacking professional training, most patients are unprepared to evaluate and comprehend any information they may receive, and furthermore, that they are too upset at being ill to be able to use the information in a manner that is rational and responsible. In effect, the profession of medicine does not view the patient as a responsible adult, but rather characterizes and treats the patient as a child (Freidson, 1970b).

The second view is that an informed patient threatens the physician's professional status and control over the therapeutic situation. An informed patient may question a medical decision or outcome and is more likely to detect professional error; by maintaining a patient as uninformed, simple protection is afforded the professional from the likelihood of uncovering mismanagement or mistakes (Skipper, Tagliacozzo, & Mauksch, 1964; Barber, 1980).

For these reasons and others, physicians appear to support and encourage patient deference. Perhaps the most widespread strategy for this is the promulgation of an image of the physician as at any moment likely to be involved in lifesaving activities (Tagliacozzo & Mauksch, 1972). Patients are reluctant to bother the physician or delay what they imagine to be critical services to other sick patients. In case after case, and regardless of how sick they are, patients express doubts about taking the doctor's time on the theory that other, more needy, patients are waiting their turn (Tuckett, Boulton, Olson, & Williams, 1985). The intensity of this belief acts as a considerable constraint on the patient's willingness to ask questions. This image of the doctor is especially evident in hospital clinics, where the atmosphere is set by alarming noises emanating from loudspeakers and intercoms, implying that a life is somewhere being saved (Quint, 1972; Davis, 1972).

Although in general patients will defer questions in consideration of the physician's busyness, occasionally patients feel they have the right to take that time. Unfortunately, the time is often simply not made available (Tagliacozzo & Mauksch, 1972), or the patient must overcome other communication-limiting strategies employed by the provider.

As a result of observing over 150 doctor visits, Svarstad (1974) identified a variety of strategies routinely employed by the physicians in her study to limit and control communication. These include:

- Turning the patient off through the intentional use of highly technical language
- Clock-watching, or watching the waiting list
- Mumbling to indicate to the patient that the physician is thinking about the medical problem and shouldn't be interrupted
- Cutting off or interrupting the patient (sometimes finishing the sentence for the patient or indicating that it would be better for the patient to speak later)
- Tuning out or ignoring the patient when he or she asks a question
- Greeting the disease instead of the person
- Executing a quick getaway rather than expressing a farewell, or simply walking out of the room without any indication to the patient that the visit has ended
- Exhibiting signs of unlikely receptivity, such as a frown or tone of sarcasm

Based on the frequency with which the physician used these strategies, visits were characterized as either hindering or facilitating communication. Under facilitating conditions about half the patients asked three or more questions; fewer than 10% of the patients under hindering conditions asked a similar number of questions. Clearly, the hindering behavior of doctors was effective in limiting patient questions. Doctors were twice as likely to employ the communication-limiting strategies when under high pressure, such as a backlogged patient waiting list, additional meetings, or other time commitments, than when they were not under any particular pressure (Svarstad, 1974).

Even under the best of circumstances, patient questions are infrequent, with no more than three or four questions asked during the typical visit (Roter, 1984). It is not surprising, then, that physicians are routinely skeptical as to whether most patients have any ideas they are interested in sharing or have questions that are unanswered (Tuckett et al., 1985). Yet it is abundantly clear from many studies that patients do indeed have ideas about their medical condition, and questions, that they want to share but do not.

KINDS OF INFORMATION PATIENTS WANT

A study asking patients what kind of information they would most like from their doctors found the highest value placed on information pertaining to prognosis, diagnosis, and origin of the condition (Kindelan & Kent, 1987). The investigators also asked the physicians treating these patients to indicate what they thought their patients would like to know. Marked discrepancies between the patients and doctors were found. Physicians dramatically underestimated patients' desire for information in the areas rated highest. These findings are consistent with prior research, which found that patients were largely uninformed about basic aspects of their condition; three-quarters of the patients did not receive even a minimal explanation of their medical condition, their prognosis, the cause of their problem, or what to expect in regard to their symptoms (Boreham & Gibson, 1978).

While the physicians underestimated the importance of diagnostic and prognostic information to patients, they overestimated the importance patients attributed to information about treatment issues, particularly drug therapy. This did not seem, however, to lead to giving consistent and complete information about drugs.

The results of a national, random survey of 1,104 persons who had received a new prescription in the preceding two weeks revealed that information given to them about their drugs was sparse. Particularly revealing were the following two findings: 35% of the patients said they didn't receive any information at all from either their doctor or pharmacist about the drugs prescribed for them; and 75% of the patients did not recall the physician telling them about possible side effects of the prescribed drugs (Miller, 1983).

Despite these obvious gaps in information about their drugs, patients were not at all active in seeking out this information. Only 2% to 4% of the patients said they asked any questions about their prescriptions while in the physician's office. It is perhaps understandable, then, that a second survey conducted with 501 primary care physicians indicated that the doctors felt that patients were satisfied with the information they were getting because few questions were asked (Miller, 1983).

Not only do doctors think patients are satisfied with the information they get, they also seem to think that patients get all the information that is good for them. Malpractice suits based on inadequate informed consent have damaged, but certainly not made obsolete, the longstanding medical tradition that favors discretion by a physician in disclosure of information to patients over the duty to tell the truth. Supported by various codes of medical ethics and by the legal doctrine of therapeutic privilege, physicians may choose to withhold relevant information from patients in cases where they believe that the information may do the patient some harm. By virtue of their expert training and knowledge, physicians can best determine what is best for their patients, or so the argument goes; the decision to disclose certain kinds of information to a patient is as much a professional decision as is the making of a diagnosis (Holder, 1970).

A leading textbook of medicine offers the following advice on what information to convey to patients:

There should be no iron-clad, inflexible rule that the patient must be told "every-thing." Few patients have the courage or faith or stoicism that the advocates of this conviction think they may or should have. . . . How much the patient is to be told will depend on his religious convictions, the wishes of his family, the state of his affairs, and his own desires and character. But even this platitude solves nothing, since it is not merely the recognition of these factors but the physician's wisdom in assessing the relative importance of each that determines how complete a discussion of the facts will best serve the interests of the patient. (Wintrobe, Thorn, Adams, Bennett, Braunwald, Isselbacher, & Petersdorf, 1970, p. 3)

The problem is that physicians and patients often disagree as to the likely outcome of disclosure, and consequently as to what is in the patient's best interest.

A study of the information preferences of patients and information-giving practices of neurologists underscores this point (Faden, Becker, Lewis, Freeman, & Faden, 1981). In general, patients preferred detailed and exten-sive disclosure of almost all risks, even when they were quite rare. Further, information about alternative therapies was highly valued by about 90% of the respondents. In contrast, the physicians indicated that they were likely to disclose only risks having a relatively high probability of occurrence; only about half of the doctors thought patients would want information about alternative therapies.

Moreover, the physicians were much more likely to agree with the view that detailed disclosure of information regarding drugs would decrease positive placebo effects, increase side effects through the power of sugges-tion, and decrease compliance. Patients expressed a completely different view. They believed more information would increase their confidence in the drug, improve their compliance, and generally serve to make them feel more comfortable with the therapy they were receiving.

Especially telling was the response to the question, "If you felt that telling a patient something about the drug would make the patient very upset and anxious, what would you do?" Sixty percent of the physicians indicated that they would inform the patient anyway, 20% would inform another member of the family, and 20% said that they would withhold the information completely. Most patients (80%) indicated that they would want to be given the information, and those who had some reservations about it indicated that they would want another member of their family to be informed. None indicated that they would want the information withheld altogether (Faden et al., 1981).

The doctor may be particularly reluctant to give information that may be bad news, ostensibly for the patient's own good, but sometimes for more self-serving reasons. In cases of poor patient prognosis, physicians have been found to withhold information for the sole purpose of patient management. In a study of fourteen families with children suffering from poliomyelitis, it was found that after two years, only one family was given a prediction of the likely clinical outcome (which was very favorable), while the remaining families (whose children were, in fact, considerably handicapped) were not told anything about what they might expect (Davis, 1972).

While the prognosis for full recovery of a child suffering from this disease is in doubt for about six weeks, the pretense of uncertainty was maintained long after the outcome was no longer uncertain. The purpose of maintaining this uncertainty was so that the physician could avoid "scenes" with patients and avoid "having to explain to and comfort them," tasks which were viewed as onerous and time-consuming. One staff member told the investigator: "We try not to tell them [parents] too much. It's better if they find out for themselves in a natural sort of way" (Davis, 1972, p. 243).

Indeed, the investigator noted that it was disheartening how, for many of the parents, this "natural sort of way" was a painfully slow and prolonged dwindling of expectations for a complete and natural recovery (Davis, 1972). Other researchers have similarly found that doctors delayed informing parents of their children's severe mental handicaps for many months and even years; again and again, patients indicated that the pain and sadness were made much worse by the wait (Quine & Pahl, 1986). Some researchers believe that health providers avoid discussions that carry bad news as protection from the sadness and difficulty that such talk is likely to create for the doctors themselves (Quint, 1972; Quine & Pahl, 1986).

While physicians may be disinclined to communicate all relevant details regarding a patient's condition, they are likely to be more conscientious about noting the particulars in the patient's medical chart. An editorial in the *New England Journal of Medicine* has proposed that legislation be passed to require that a complete and unexpurgated copy of all medical records, both inpatient and outpatient, be given to patients routinely and automatically (Shenkin & Warner, 1973). Others have argued for at least open access to medical records (Stevens & MacKay, 1977; Golodetz, Ruess, & Machaus, 1976) or even for having patients coauthor the medical record (Fischback, Bayog, Needle, & Delbanco, 1980).

These authors argue that the medical chart can fill the gaps in communication between doctor and patient, act as an educational tool for patients, reduce suspicion that the physician is keeping something from patients, and enable patients to act more autonomously in making judgments and choices about their care. As we shall see in Chapter 9, the medical chart may be just the tool that is needed to help patients and doctors talk more productively to one another. However, sharing of the medical chart is infrequent and information is generally tightly controlled. The consequences of information control appear far-reaching, affecting the therapeutic relationship in very basic ways.

Several investigators have suggested that the tradition of provider control of information contributes to patients' misunderstanding of their role in the relationship, encouraging a misleading passivity in which patients appear to wait for the provider to take the initiative in explanations, while the physician, on the other hand, takes the patient's reserve as an indication of disinterest or incompetence (Cartwright, 1964; Pratt, Seligmann, & Reader, 1957).

This has been portrayed as a communication-limiting cycle that works as follows:

When a doctor perceives the patient as rather poorly informed, he considers the tremendous difficulties of translating his knowledge into language the patient can understand along with the dangers of frightening the patient. Therefore, he avoids involving himself in an elaborate discussion with the patient; the patient, in turn, reacts dully to this limited information, either asking uninspired questions or refraining from questioning the doctor at all, thus reinforcing the doctor's view that the patient is ill-equipped to comprehend his problem. This further reinforces the doctor's tendency to skirt discussions of the problem. Lacking guidance by the doctor, the patient performs at a low level; hence the doctor rates his capacities as even lower than they are. (Pratt, Seligmann, & Reader, 1957, p. 1281)

Some support for the idea of the communication-limiting cycle is derived from the finding that patients who received some explanation from the physician tended to respond with more questions than did those patients who were not given any explanation.

One conclusion that may be drawn from this is that physicians set the tone of the interaction and have primary control over patient participation in the medical visit; patients are more active when the physician provides at least a minimal framework of information within which the patient can arrange thoughts and formulate questions. Not all questions, however, are derived from technical knowledge. It is easy to imagine that personal experience, anxiety, fright, and the observation of others provide a basis for patient questioning. Patients are not dependent on physician-provided explanations of illness to formulate the kinds of questions described above. Yet, patients do not ask many questions of any kind.

The earliest studies in this area found that patients seldom made forceful demands for information from their physicians, although a substantial proportion of patients would frankly admit to an interviewer that they would like more information about some fundamental aspects of their condition (Kutner,

1972; Reader, Pratt, & Mudd, 1957). Some thirty years later, little seems to have changed. Tuckett and his associates (Tuckett et al., 1985) conducted in-depth interviews with ninety-eight patients, in which they were asked if they had any specific doubts or questions during their medical visits that they did not mention to the doctor. Three-quarters of the patients said yes.

The majority of the patients did not ask questions because the patients felt afraid of the doctor's reaction. Fear of humiliation by the doctor was the most common deterrent from asking questions. Patients expressed dread of having the doctor think badly of them or misunderstand their motivation for questioning. They were anxious that the doctor not think that they were second-guessing his or her judgment. Further, few patients thought that their doctors actually wanted them to question them, and patients felt an urgency about the time they were taking from the doctor's really needy patients. Feeling hurried clearly interfered with the patient's ability to gather his or her thoughts and clearly articulate questions. For these patients, the lack of question asking was far more likely to reflect a lack of skill in clearly articulating ideas or questions than lack of interest.

Lack of patient skill in question asking has been observed in other studies. In fact, one researcher observed that the main communication problem physicians faced was the patients' inability to express themselves clearly. In response to an open-ended opportunity to speak, patients just ran out of words; the doctor then took the floor to prevent an uneasy silence (Hughs, 1982).

Perhaps, then, patients need help in developing their question-asking skills. Just such a study was conducted by Roter (1977). Half the patients, who were attending a community health clinic, were randomly assigned to an experiment to increase the number of questions they asked during their medical visit. The other half of the patients were given a session on a topic unrelated to question asking. Each of the patients in the experimental group talked with an interviewer in the waiting room for about ten minutes immediately before seeing the doctor. The focus of the discussion was on questions the patient might want to ask the doctor. The interviewer facilitated the process by going through a list of common questions that were likely to be relevant. The patients were offered help in articulating their questions and given an opportunity to rehearse their questions. Finally, they were given a supportive message underscoring the importance of asking questions.

The average number of questions asked by these patients was twice that asked by patients in the other group, and the questions were in medically relevant areas. It is indeed possible to increase patient questions. However, it should be noted that this increased number was still less than two questions per patient.

Table 6.1
A Guide to Asking Questions

Asking questions is a very important part of your visit to the doctor. By asking questions your doctor can help clear up doubts, concerns, or worries. It is an important way in which you can get things straight. Don't just worry about something, *ask!*

A. DIAGNOSIS

Has the doctor told you what your problem is, that is, has the doctor told you what the diagnosis is?

Do you think this is correct, or that something else or something more is the problem?

B. ETIOLOGY

Do you know what caused your problem?

C. PROGNOSIS

Have you discussed the seriousness of this problem with the doctor?

Do you know how long your problem will last?

Do you know how long it will be until there is an improvement?

Are you worried that it will come back or get worse?

Are you worried about how this problem may be affecting your health in the long run?

D. TREATMENT

Do you know how the doctor proposes to treat your problem?

Do you understand why the doctor thinks this treatment is the best?

Is there any other kind of treatment that you think might work?

E. MEDICATIONS

Has your doctor prescribed any medication for you?

If so:

Do you know the name of the medication?

Do you know how the medicine helps you?

Do you know when to take the medicine, for instance, do you know what to do if you miss a dose—do you take two when you remember or just skip the missed dose?

If the drug is to be taken every four hours, does that mean you should waken during the night to take your dose?

Do you know what possible side effects are associated with the medicine, for example, is it likely to make you drowsy or nauseated?

Is the drug likely to interact with any over-the-counter, nonprescription drugs you may be taking, or with alcohol?

Table 6.1 (continued)

F. TESTS

Has your doctor ordered any tests?

If so, are you sure of the purpose of the tests ordered and what the results will be used for?

G. LIFESTYLE

Has the doctor suggested a change in any lifestyle habits such as smoking, drinking alcohol, exercise, weight, or diet?

If so:

Do you know how much change is needed to make a difference?

Were you given any hints about how to make these changes easier?

H. PREVENTION

Do you know what you can do to prevent this problem in the future?

Do you know if your problem runs in the family?

If so, do you know what you can do to help others from developing this problem?

When patients ask questions, their doctors virtually always provide them with answers (Roter, 1977; Svarstad, 1974; Boreham & Gibson, 1978). Further, patients who are more verbally active during the visit by offering their own explanations or thoughts about their condition, asking questions, or expressing doubts are treated differently than patients who are not as active (Tuckett et al., 1985). Generally, the more active patients receive the kind of practical information needed to help them make decisions. Clearly, this can make a dramatic difference in how much information the patient takes away from the visit.

In contrast to the conclusion that the physician determines the nature of the interaction by providing or withholding information, it may well be the patient who influences the interaction by indicating the desire for a more active or passive stance in the relationship. Because question asking is the most usual indicator of patient activity in the interaction, physicians may take the expression of a question to indicate a desire for greater participation. As a result, these patients could receive more detailed explanations of their illness, and be more of a partner in the communication process.

To help lay readers when they become patients, we offer a guide to asking questions (Table 6.1). It is based on our own past work and the work of others, notably David Tuckett and his colleagues in England (1985).

NOT ALL PATIENTS WANT TO ASK QUESTIONS

Some 15% of the patients interviewed in the English study by Tuckett and colleagues (1985) indicated that they had not asked questions of their doctors. These patients said that they were not interested—they felt knowing about medical matters was "not for them." The lack of question asking may reflect lack of confidence and skill for many patients—but for some patients it may reflect true avoidance of or resistance to information.

Social psychologists have argued that some individuals may benefit more than others from being highly informed or involved in their own treatment, and that for some patients, detailed information may actually increase anxiety through information overload (Mills & Krantz, 1979). For instance, Miller and associates (Miller & Mangan, 1983) found that it was useful to classify patients as information-avoiders or information-seekers to determine their psychophysiological response to varying levels of information while undergoing a painful medical procedure. The researchers found that patients' level of anxiety was lower when the level of information given to them was consistent with their coping style; information-avoiders did better with less information and information-seekers did better with more.

Additional insight into the distinction between avoiders and seekers is provided by Steptoe and colleagues (Steptoe, Sutcliffe, Allen, & Coombes, 1991). The investigators found that while all patients who reported that they understood little about their condition desired additional information, information-avoiders generally reported higher understanding of their condition and greater satisfaction with doctor-patient communication than information-seekers. However, scores on objective knowledge tests were lower for the avoiders. The authors conclude that information-avoiders report a better understanding of their condition, not because of superior factual knowledge but "because their coping style led them to avoid further direct information that might highlight their predicament" (Steptoe et al., 1991, p. 628). Despite better understanding, information-seekers were nonetheless less satisfied with communication and felt there was more to know about their condition that they would like the doctor to share with them.

THE TWO-WAY FLOW OF INFORMATION

As is evident in this chapter, most researchers have conceptualized the informative event as driven largely by an assumption of a unidirectional flow of information from physician to patient—either stimulated by patient questions or as information spontaneously given by the provider to the patient. However, there is a broader perspective on informative events in the medical visit that challenges the assumption of unidirectional flow. Effective information exchange is an interactive, two-way process, and within these exchanges the usefulness of the information a patient gets is very often contingent on the information the patient gives.

Patients spend most of their time during the medical visit providing information to physicians—largely in response to physicians' questions (mostly closed-ended) about the medical condition. But this kind of information is incomplete. Giving patients the opportunity to tell their story in an open manner, with minimal direction by the physician, can increase both provider and patient understanding of the patient's condition and his or her experience. The reflection and insight that can arise from the telling of the story can move the level of exchange to a deeper and more meaningful interaction.

Another important type of information that patients only infrequently share with the physician, and about which physicians infrequently inquire, is their explanatory framework. This is patients' interpretations of how and why they are sick, what will make them better, and what they hope the doctor can do for them. This kind of insight can provide the physician with a starting point for meaningful exchange. Knowing where patients are in terms of their beliefs and theories is essential if the provider hopes to attach relevance to the information given to the patient. Otherwise, information giving in the medical dialogue can be reduced to "two parallel monologues," in which patient and physician are talking at cross-purposes and in two different languages (Mishler, 1984).

Moreover, information exchange conveys more than just substantive meaning. Research suggests that patients attribute positive affective motivation to a physician who is informative; the physician who takes time to inform patients fully is seen as sincere, concerned, interested, and dedicated (Roter, Hall, & Katz, 1988). There is also evidence that physicians attribute positive characteristics to patients who are more verbally active in their visit, viewing them as more interested, concerned about their health, and intelligent.

Where do we go from here? One suggestion is that it is not sufficient simply to encourage physicians to be more informative or to train patients to ask more questions. That view takes doctor-patient interaction out of its context and strips it of much of its dynamic productivity. Rather, it is important to appreciate the tremendous power of permitting patients to orient the physician to their "lifeworld"—to tell their story and share their experiences, understanding, theories, and concerns about their health (Mishler, 1984). It is this process that is informative to both the patient and the physician, and from which important questions will freely arise and comprehensible information will emerge.

REFERENCES

Barber, B. (1980). *Informed consent in medical therapy and research*. New Brunswick, N.J.: Rutgers University Press.

Boreham, P., & Gibson, D. (1978). The informative process in private medical consultations: A preliminary investigation. *Social Science & Medicine, 12*, 409–416.

Cartwright, A. (1964). *Human relations and hospital care*. London: Routledge & Kegan Paul.

Christy, N. P. (1979). English is our second language. *New England Journal of Medicine, 300*, 979–981.

Davis, F. (1972). Uncertainty in medical prognosis, clinical and functional. In Freidson, E., & Lorber, J. (Eds.), *Medical men and their work: A sociological reader*. Chicago: Aldine Atherton.

Faden, R., Becker, C., Lewis, C., Freeman, J., & Faden, A. (1981). Disclosure of information to patients in medical care. *Medical Care, 19*, 718–733.

Fischback, R. L., Bayog, A. S., Needle, A., & Delbanco, T. L. (1980). The patient and practitioner as co-authors of the medical record. *Patient Counseling and Health Education, 2*, 1–5.

Freidson, E. (1970b). *Professional dominance*. Chicago: Aldine Press.

Golodetz, A., Ruess, J., & Machaus, R. L. (1976). The right to know: Giving the patient his medical record. *Archives of Physical and Medical Rehabilitation, 57*, 78–81.

Holder, A. R. (1970). Informed consent: Its evolution. *Journal of the American Medical Association, 214*, 1181–1182.

Hughs, D. (1982). Control in medical consultation: The organizing talk in a situation where co-participants have differential competence. *Sociology, 16*, 359–376.

Kindelan, K., & Kent, G. (1987). Concordance between patients' information preferences and general practitioners' perceptions. *Psychology and Health, 1*, 399–409.

Korsch, B. M., Gozzi, E. K., & Francis, V. (1968). Gaps in doctor-patient communication. *Pediatrics, 42*, 855–871.

Kutner, B. (1972). Surgeons and their patients: A study in social perception. In Jaco, E. G. (Ed.), *Patients, physicians and illness*. New York: The Free Press.

McKinlay, J. B. (1975). Who is really ignorant—Physician or patient? *Journal of Health and Social Behavior, 16*, 3–11.

Miller, R. W. (1983). Doctors, patients don't communicate. *FDA Consumer*. HHS publication no. (FDA) 83–1102.

Miller, S. M., & Mangan, C. E. (1983). Interacting effects of information and coping style in adapting to gynecologic stress: Should the doctor tell all? *Journal of Personality and Social Psychology, 45*, 223–236.

Mills, R. T., & Krantz, D. (1979). Information choice and reactions to stress: A field experiment in a blood bank with laboratory analogue. *Journal of Personality and Social Psychology, 37*, 608–620.

Mishler, E. G. (1984). *The discourse of medicine: Dialectics of medical interviews.* Norwood, N.J.: Ablex.

Pratt, L., Seligmann, A., & Reader, G. (1957). Physicians' views on the level of medical information among patients. *American Journal of Public Health, 47,* 1277–1283.

Quine, L., & Pahl, J. (1986). First diagnosis of severe mental handicap: Characteristics of unsatisfactory encounters between doctors and parents. *Social Science & Medicine, 22,* 53–62.

Quint, J. (1972). Institutionalized practices of information control. In Freidson, E., & Lorber, J. (Eds.), *Medical men and their work: A sociological reader.* Chicago: Aldine Atherton.

Reader, G. S., Pratt, L., & Mudd, M. C. (1957). What do patients expect from their doctors? *Modern Hospital, 89,* 88–91.

Roter, D. (1977). Patient participation in the patient-provider interaction: The effects of patient question asking on the quality of interaction, satisfaction, and compliance. *Health Education Monographs, 5,* 281–315.

Roter, D. L. (1984). Patient question asking in physician-patient interaction. *Health Psychology, 3,* 395–409.

Roter, D. L., Hall, J. A., & Katz, N. R. (1988). Patient-physician communication: A descriptive summary of the literature. *Patient Education and Counseling, 12,* 99–119.

Shenkin, B., & Warner, D. (1973). Giving the patient his medical record: A proposal to improve the system. *New England Journal of Medicine, 289,* 688–691.

Skipper, J. K., Tagliacozzo, D. L., & Mauksch, H. O. (1964). Some possible consequences of limited communication between patients and hospital functionaries. *Journal of Health and Human Behavior, 6,* 34.

Steptoe, A., Sutcliffe, I., Allen, B., & Coombes, C. (1991). Satisfaction with communication, medical knowledge, and coping style in patients with metastatic cancer. *Social Science & Medicine, 32,* 627–632.

Stevens, D. P., & MacKay, C. R. (1977). What happens when hospitalized patients see their records? *Annals of Internal Medicine, 86,* 474–477.

Svarstad, B. L. (1974). *The doctor-patient encounter: An observational study of communication and outcome.* Doctoral dissertation, University of Wisconsin, Madison.

Tagliacozzo, D. L., & Mauksch, H. O. (1972). The patient's view of the patient role. In Jaco, E. G. (Ed.), *Patients, physicians and illness.* New York: The Free Press.

Tuckett, D., Boulton, M., Olson, C., & Williams, A. (1985). *Meetings between experts.* New York: Tavistock Publications.

Wintrobe, M. M., Thorn, G. W., Adams, R. D., Bennett, I. L., Jr., Braunwald, E., Isselbacher, K. J., & Petersdorf, R. G. (Eds.) (1970). *Harrison's principles of internal medicine.* New York: McGraw-Hill.

Part III
Prospects for Improved Talk

7

Talk and the Quality of Care

One can think of the quality of care as residing, ultimately, in the health of the patient, and some experts on quality do define it that way. But health, or lack of it, is determined by many factors besides the nature of the care actually rendered to the patient. Stress, for example, weakens the immune system, and economic factors also influence people's health in a variety of ways. A low-income mother has trouble affording medications for her children; poorly educated people may not fully understand the need for regular care; a breadwinner in a minimum-wage job puts his or her job at risk by taking time off to visit the doctor. Medical care providers may have little or no influence in these areas.

Because a person's state of health has many causes, most research on the quality of care focuses on the process rather than the outcome of care. Process refers to those things that providers actually do, and fail to do, in the clinical situation. This approach recognizes that doing the "right" thing doesn't guarantee a well or even an improved patient, but it at least permits systematic study of what the health care providers have done for a patient.

Although there is often uncertainty in the profession, even disagreement, over what constitutes appropriate medical care, standards have been developed for the handling of many medical conditions; some examples are ear infection, acute myocardial infarction (heart attack), diabetes, chronic bronchitis, gonorrhea, burns, and urinary tract infection. The standards set for such conditions typically cover certain facts from the medical history and physical examination, the adequacy of the diagnostic process, and the development of plans for managing the illness. By applying these standards to transcriptions of visits or to the content of medical records, researchers can come up with scores describing how well a doctor performs.

The vast majority of studies on quality of care are based entirely on technical criteria such as these and ignore completely the manner in which care is delivered, the humaneness of the provider, and the adequacy of the physician as a teacher. Very likely, these aspects of care are accorded lower priority by some in the medical profession—considered just "bedside manners." Alternatively, it is sometimes believed that although interpersonal aspects of care are important, it is not possible to develop standards for them, or that it is not even necessary to do so since a doctor just naturally knows how to handle this side of his or her role.

We think these beliefs are wrong. As every patient knows, there are doctors who are woefully inadequate interpersonally and others who inspire such confidence and such a sense of well-being that simply seeing them or hearing their voice makes one feel better. Furthermore, enough knowledge is available so that standards could be developed in this domain, and studies have shown that interpersonal skills can be both taught and measured.

But because of prevailing beliefs, researchers have only occasionally developed criteria for good interpersonal care, which might include greeting patients appropriately, offering appropriate amounts of reassurance or empathy, or legitimizing the patients' expression of psychosocial concerns. Most studies that measure interpersonal behavior simply describe what is done, without going the next step of prescribing what should be done.

There is no debate, of course, that interpersonal care rests on the talk between doctors and patients, for this is true almost by definition. Talk (both verbal and nonverbal) is the medium through which they get to know one another, negotiate their roles, and communicate their feelings, expectations, and intentions.

Yet talk is almost always deficient in one way or another. Studies document, for example, low levels of concordance between doctors and patients on what the patient's problem is and how it came about, even after they have supposedly reached an understanding. It is as though the two speak different languages or live in different worlds (Mishler, 1984). This lack of mutual understanding can rest on mismatched frames of reference as well as inadequate talk. In a study conducted in an HMO in Providence, Rhode Island, a sample of doctors and their elderly patients were both asked to rate the patient's overall current health. From an examination of relations between these ratings and other health indicators, it was evident that overall health meant different things to doctor and patient (Hall, Epstein, & McNeil, 1989). The patients' ratings were more holistic—related to both their functional abilities and their emotional distress, as well as the number and complexity of their medical problems. The doctors' ratings were more narrowly defined and closely related to medical diagnoses.

We have been trying to illustrate the obvious role of talk in the interpersonal side of care. But there is a fine line between the interpersonal and technical that occurs during the transmission of information. The patient who successfully communicates feelings, needs, and values (usually relegated to the interpersonal domain of communication) is also building the database that the physician will use to make a diagnosis (a technical aspect of care).

We would go even further and state that the entire technical side of medicine rests mainly on talk. This becomes especially evident when there can be no communication—when the patient is unconscious. In that circumstance every aspect of care becomes more difficult and prone to error, and physicians signal their dependence on talk by seeking out family members or witnesses to supply some of the missing dialogue. But unconscious patients are relatively rare, and in the great majority of medical encounters talk is the basis of decision and action, as well as motivation on both sides.

RESEARCH ON QUALITY OF CARE

A brief description of research on the quality of medical care will serve two purposes in this chapter: first, to illustrate the relation of talk to quality, and, second, to build our argument that change is possible in doctor-patient interactions.

A study of physicians in western Pennsylvania sheds some light on this topic (Roter, Hall, & Katz, 1987; Hall, Roter, & Katz, 1987; Roter & Hall, 1987; Hall & Roter, 1988; Wang, Terry, Flynn, Williamson, Green, & Faden, 1979). Each physician, out of a total of forty-eight, was audiotaped while interviewing and examining two middle-aged patients in ordinary office visits. One patient had emphysema, the other chronic bronchitis.

The visits were not quite ordinary, in that the two patients were simulated patients hired by the researchers to pay visits to these doctors. They actually had the medical conditions they described, and they were coached to present consistent histories and complaints to one doctor after another, so that the researchers could compare the doctors' performances. The researchers developed, with the help of a panel of experts on lung disease, a long checklist of things that would constitute high-quality care for each simulated patient. Each doctor's performance was scored in terms of the proportion of correct actions taken. We also scored the interaction of the visit by applying the Roter Interaction Analysis Scheme (RIAS) to all talk of the visit. This system codes every statement into mutually exclusive and exhaustive categories to enable a frequency count of every verbal behavior that occurs during the medical dialogue.

Table 7.1
Performance of Physicians in Western Pennsylvania

Measure	Average Score (%)
Proficiency in terms of asking appropriate closed (yes-no or highly focused) questions	50
Proficiency in terms of asking appropriate open-ended questions	26
Proficiency in terms of eliciting key facts from the patient	55
Proficiency in terms of giving the patient general information pertinent to his condition	15
Proficiency in terms of employing teaching strategies for patient education (such as asking the patient to repeat facts)	24
Proficiency in terms of diagnosis, tests, and/or treatments recommended (clinical expertise)	53

Source: Unpublished data from Hall, Roter, and Katz (1987) and Roter, Hall, and Katz (1987).

In Table 7.1 we show how the doctors scored. Generally, they achieved less than half of what the experts said they should. One can, of course, argue that the experts were being unrealistically strict. But even if we leniently add another 20% to the average scores, to compensate for any excesses of strictness, performance is still far from perfect. Even if we add 40%—this is very lenient indeed—the average score is still only 77%.

Of the six kinds of proficiency shown in Table 7.1, all but the last are obviously based on the talk between doctor and patient. But even the last kind of proficiency, quality of clinical decision making, is also heavily dependent on the quality of talk, for the doctor's knowledge of medicine cannot be applied without knowledge of the particulars of a given case. The data of this study support this point of view, for proficiency in clinical decision making was strongly correlated with the "talking" proficiencies (the first five in the table).

Indeed, we also found that the content analysis of the interaction, that is, the frequency counts of physicians' verbal behavior, was strongly related to proficiency. The more information in general (and biomedical information in particular) and counseling the doctors gave, and the fewer closed-ended questions and directions, the more proficient the doctors were according to the expert-generated checklist. We also found that the doctors in our study who scored higher on a knowledge test of chronic obstructive disease were more likely to engage in these same verbal behaviors than less proficient doctors.

But perhaps these results showing disappointing performance are not typical. It is, after all, a small sample of doctors in rural practice settings. And the results may be misleading because of the artificiality of the simulated patient methodology.

Dutch researchers designed a quality of care study that addressed these major limitations in our own work. Bensing (1991) conducted a study in which 103 hypertension visits were assessed for quality by having videotapes of the encounters assessed by a group of twelve trained physicians. The physicians independently rated the videotapes for three dimensions of quality of care. These included: (1) the technical-medical dimension, summarized by a nationally accepted treatment protocol on the detection and treatment of hypertension, as well as some general aspects of quality such as the avoidance of superfluous treatment; (2) the psychosocial dimension, including the degree to which the physician responded to and investigated the nonsomatic aspects of hypertension, the psychosocial concerns of patients, as well as the background and consequences of the condition; and (3) the doctor-patient relationship, reflecting the manner in which the doctor dealt with the patient and the extent to which an open, secure, and workable relationship was established.

Scoring on the three dimensions was done on a ten-point scale, and the physician-judges showed considerable consistency in their assessments. The average assessment of the quality of technical-medical treatment was 6.5, with a range between 4.6 and 7.6. Psychosocial treatment averaged 6.2, with a range from 3.3 to 8.0, and the quality of the doctor-patient relationship averaged 6.6, with a range from 3.8 to 8.1.

In order to investigate the relationship between the clinical judgment of the physician-judges and the talk of the medical visit, Bensing analyzed the videotapes using RIAS, the same interaction process system used in our study of physicians in western Pennsylvania. The results were quite dramatic, with many similarities to our own findings. A remarkably high percentage of the variation (ranging from 59% to 70%) in the physician-judges' quality assessments was explained by interaction analysis. Particularly important were positive affect ratings (i.e., interest, warmth, and attentiveness), as well as specific categories reflecting the giving of medical information by physicians, and more socioemotional categories such as reflecting, paraphrasing, and showing agreement.

Taken together these two studies present a convincing argument relating communication skills to technical quality of care. It is especially convincing that similar conclusions were reached despite differences in setting and methodology. We believe that more studies of this kind are absolutely critical. As this base of research continues, we believe that they will lay the foundation for communication-based certification and evaluation of physician performance.

A more common approach to assessing quality is represented by the work of a group of Boston researchers, in which the quality of care given by several hundred doctors and nurse practitioners was assessed by medical record review (Palmer, Strain, Maurer, Rothrock, & Thompson, 1984; Palmer, Strain, Maurer, & Thompson, 1984). The practices they stuied, sixteen in all, were both adult and pediatric, and were situated in both teaching hospitals associated with major medical schools and neighborhood health centers that were associated with teaching hospitals. Care associated with teaching hospitals is, generally speaking, quite good.

Medical charts were examined and scored according to a complex set of quality standards. Each of the medical tasks examined, such as follow-up of abnormal blood test results or conducting a well-child examination, had a set of such standards or criteria. For example, for follow-up of low red blood cell count, the medical care provider was supposed to repeat the test, find out whether the problem was iron deficiency, find out whether there was internal bleeding, and do a rectal examination, among other things.

Table 7.2 shows the findings for adults, in terms of the percentage of patients whose care was fully adequate, that is, for whom all standards applying to their particular condition were met. In order not to penalize providers who had good justification for not doing something that was on the "do" list, all instances of apparent deficiencies in care were reviewed by a physician at the site to be doubly sure the failures of care were really without justification.

For the blood-sugar task, performance was very good (94% of cases were appropriately handled), but for the other three tasks large numbers of patients received care that was deficient in one or more ways. For the pediatric tasks many oversights were also found, some of which we reproduce in Table 7.3.

It is important, in reviewing this study, to know that the standards being used to evaluate these providers' performance were not esoteric or unacceptably strict. In fact, before the study was done the physician leaders in these

Table 7.2

Performance of Medical Providers in Boston Study, for Adult Medical Conditions

Medical Task	Cases with Fully Adequate Care (%)
Follow-up of low red blood cell count	69
Cancer screening for women (Pap smear and breast exam)	69
Follow-up of high blood sugar	94
Monitoring of drug regimen for patients with congestive heart failure	58

Source: Adapted from Table 2 of Palmer, Strain, Maurer, Rothrock, & Tompson (1984).

same medical practices discussed the standards and indicated very high rates of agreement with them. It is simply quite evident that in actual medical practice, both doctors and nurse practitioners fail surprisingly often to live up to their good intentions. The care they render is more flawed than their formal knowledge of accepted practice would lead one to expect.

Although we can only speculate on what accounts for this, talk could play a significant role in several of the results. Cancer screening in women, especially the breast exam, may involve a delicate negotiation between patient and physician. Some women are reluctant to request these exams at all, especially from male physicians, who may themselves be uneasy about them. The accomplishment of these exams may require confidence of the patient in the physician as well as a physician who takes time to discover and discuss the patient's values and reactions.

Another task, monitoring of the drug regimen for patients with congestive heart failure, is essentially talk: does the physician find out what the patient is taking and how he or she is faring with the drug? For some of the other tasks in Tables 7.2 and 7.3, failures of talk could also underlie failures of performance. A doctor might be less likely to follow up on abnormal test results if he or she knows less about the patient's history, or if the patient takes no initiative to inquire about the result and what it means. And a doctor conducting a well-child exam may be less likely to measure height and weight if the parent makes no request or inquiry along these lines.

Table 7.3
Performance of Medical Providers in Boston Study, for Pediatric Tasks

Medical Task and Criterion	Rate of Successful Performance (%)
Well-child care:	
Recorded height?	75
Recorded weight?	82
Checked for anemia (if needed)?	84
Checked for lead in blood?	68
Ear infection:	
Described tympanic membrane (eardrum)?	62
Scheduled follow-up visit?	86

Source: Adapted from Tables 2 and 3 of Palmer, Strain, Maurer, & Thompson (1984).

A 1988 report in the *Lancet* (Domenighetti, Luraschi, Casabianca, Gutzwiller, Spinelli, Pedrinis, & Repetto, 1988) underscores the importance of information about quality of care, and how patients may use it. Earlier research by these investigators found that the hysterectomy rate for a studied region in Switzerland was very high and increasing at an alarming rate— more than doubling in the five-year period from 1977–82. Moreover, the rates of hysterectomy were highly correlated with the number of gynecologists and surgical beds rather than the logically expected population parameters such as morbidity, mortality, and sociodemographics.

To publicize their findings, the authors began a mass media campaign lasting some six months using newspapers, radio and radio call-in programs, and television to disseminate the results of their study and raise the "hysterectomy question." Over the five years after the campaign (1982–86), the annual rate of hysterectomy per 100,000 women decreased by 25.8%, compared with a 1% increase in the German-speaking Swiss comparison city of Bern. (Both cities had comparable hysterectomy rates for the five years prior to the study's beginning in 1982.) The researchers conclude that their media campaign was instrumental in disturbing the patient-doctor relationship, on the one hand by disseminating to patients information about medical procedures usually available only to the medical profession, and, on the other hand, by increasing professional accountability to patients about indications for surgery.

We are not suggesting that the burden should be on patients to oversee doctor performance, or that patients should be held responsible when doctors do not follow accepted practice standards. But we do suggest that patients and doctors, through their communication, create a climate that can foster or inhibit quality of care, and that an inquisitive, involved patient who makes wishes known could easily remind the doctor of things that might otherwise be forgotten, ignored, or postponed.

Some patient preferences may be at odds with recommended medical practice. It is possible that some of the women forgoing a hysterectomy could have benefited from the operation, but because of suspicion and misunderstanding of the appropriate circumstances for this surgery, they resisted their doctor's recommendation.

A more common scenario is likely to be that a woman forgoes a breast or pelvic exam because the procedure is embarrassing, and she makes it quite clear to her male physician that the exam would make her uncomfortable. But if the matter rested here, we would fault the physician. The physician has a duty to try to change his patients' attitudes by teaching the benefits of early cancer detection, or suggesting that a female physician or nurse perform the exam. We do not claim that all failures of technical practice stem from faulty communication, but we think many do.

Another study, this one on general internists in Maryland, Virginia, and Washington, D.C., also provides revealing information on the quality of care (Sanazaro & Worth, 1985). Eight diagnoses (for example, arthritis, hypertension, and angina pectoris) were selected. In this rather complex study, three groups of physicians participated—those whose performance was being studied, a national panel of experts who determined what good care should be, and a group of physicians who read summaries of actual patient cases of the first group of doctors and rated the adequacy of the care the doctors provided. Two aspects of care were examined: whether the doctor adequately substantiated the diagnosis before starting treatment, and whether the doctor provided adequate management of the condition once it was diagnosed.

Scores were always higher for substantiating the diagnosis than for therapeutic management, and scores were higher for patients who were hospitalized than for those who were seen in doctors' offices. In the hospital, 4% of the cases were judged to be substandard, with the worst being diabetes mellitus (6%) and acute bacterial pneumonia (8%). In offices, a full 13% of cases received substandard care, with the worst being diabetes mellitus (17%) and hypertension (15%).

VARIATION IN CARE

Low average levels of physician performance certainly indicate that care should be improved. However, another kind of information is equally important: how uniform is care, irrespective of its overall level? Finding out about variation in quality is important because if care does vary, one's immediate question is why? Is it just inexplicable, random variation? If not, what can account for it? Does a particular kind of doctor render excellent care, or does a particular kind of patient tend to get better care? Are certain activities or behaviors, or forms of communication between doctors and patients, associated with better care?

Care is highly variable, that we can say with certainty. In the study of doctors in Pennsylvania who were visited by simulated patients, we calculated quality of care scores for the different doctors by averaging their performance in a given category over the two patients they saw (Hall, Roter, & Katz, 1987). Thus, a doctor's score would be 0% if he did none of the recommended things in either visit, and 100% if he did all of them in both visits. The variation between doctors was extreme, to say the least. For asking appropriate closed-ended questions (questions usually answered by yes or no), performance scores ranged from 36% to 72%—that is, the worst-scoring doctor earned only 36% for this category and the best earned 72%. For eliciting important facts from the patient, performance scores ranged from 9% to 85%. And for expertise in clinical judgments, performance scores ranged from 33% to 71%.

Variation was also striking in the Boston study of sixteen group practices (Palmer Studies dated 1984b). Rather than presenting differences between providers, Palmer and her colleagues first averaged all the scores within a medical practice and then displayed the range of those averages across medical practices (again 100% would be perfect performance). For follow-up of low red blood cell count, the medical practices' average performance scores ranged from 43% to 81%. For cancer screening in women, the scores of the medical practices ranged from 55% to 84%. For follow-up of high blood sugar, the scores ranged from 87% to 100%. And for monitoring drugs in people with heart failure, the scores ranged from 44% to 68%.

The study of internists around Maryland and Virginia also showed variation between doctors (Sanazaro & Worth, 1985). Although quite a few delivered perfect care to all their patients who were studied, some provided substandard care (as defined by the researchers) to a quarter or more of their patients. If technical performance, for which physicians are trained in medical school, is highly variable, then we would expect the more interpersonal aspects of care, which are barely trained, to vary even more. The forty-three doctors in Pennsylvania seem to confirm such a prediction. The number of statements made by the doctor to counsel the patient about health or lifestyle ranged from 1 to 130, and the number of positive (approving or encouraging) statements by the doctor ranged from 2 to 60 (Hall, Roter, & Katz, 1987).

VARIATION IN TEST-ORDERING AND DRUG PRESCRIBING BEHAVIOR

We have talked at length about variations in technical quality and communication. But other variations have been found that are also troubling. One might assume, for example, that it is obvious to doctors when they should order blood, urine, or imaging (such as X-ray) tests as an aid to diagnosis, and that these decisions depend on the particulars of a given patient case. Not so. Variations in testing habits are great—between doctors within a given facility, between medical specialties, between different ways the delivery of care is organized (such as private, fee-for-service physicians versus those salaried in an HMO), between different regions of the country, and between the United States and England. Sometimes different physicians or care settings show fivefold or even tenfold differences in testing rates (Epstein & McNeil, 1987).

Unfortunately, the relation between how many and what kinds of tests are done by physicians, on the one hand, and the quality of overall care rendered to patients, on the other, is largely unknown. But research does indicate that very often the tests that are ordered are inappropriate (Epstein & McNeil, 1987). Because tests account for a large proportion of health care costs, there is much pressure on physicians, at least in certain settings, to cut down their rates of test ordering.

HMOs, in particular, stand to gain economically by such steps, since they take in a fixed dollar amount per patient. A provocative study found that HMOs and fee-for-service medical practices had similar rates of ordering low-cost tests such as blood counts and urine tests, but differed significantly on the high-cost, high-profit tests such as electrocardiograms. The fee-for-service physicians used more of the expensive tests (Epstein, Begg, & McNeil, 1986). Often, fee-for-service physicians, especially those in large groups, have a financial incentive to order more tests—if they perform the tests on-site, they make a profit on them. Because doctors often make a profit on tests, they would resist steps taken by outsiders to limit test use. Some evidence suggests, for example, that if insurance companies were to reimburse physicians less per test, as a disincentive to perform so many tests, physicians would just order more tests so as to maintain their previous income (Epstein & McNeil, 1987).

The tendency of doctors to order a great many diagnostic tests may reflect the technological imperative of modern medicine, and also may be a response to the threat of malpractice suits. Either way, there is much concern over it, both for economic reasons and because of risks to patients (not all tests are perfectly safe, and false positive results can lead to unneeded further treatment). A number of studies have experimented with various kinds of incentives and forms of pressure to reduce the volume of testing, especially in hospitals.

Although there is good reason to discourage overuse of diagnostic tests, our analysis in terms of talk between doctors and patients would suggest that across-the-board efforts may not get at the heart of the problem. Often, too many or inappropriate tests are ordered simply because the doctor does not have enough pertinent information to make better-targeted decisions. This lack could stem from insufficient questioning by the doctor or withholding of information by the patient (on purpose or accidentally). The typical line of yes-no questions employed by physicians can certainly result in inappropriate orders for tests, if this questioning closes off the patient's full story and leads the doctor into testing hypotheses that turn out to be wrong.

Testing is only one area that shows extremes of variation; drug-prescribing practice is another. Close to two-thirds of all medical visits in the United States result in the prescribing of one or more drugs. However, there is wide variation in physicians' practices, and the appropriateness of many prescriptions may be questioned (Hemminki, 1975).

The variation in appropriateness of drug-prescribing behaviors is not random. Some kinds of doctors are more proficient in this area than others. For instance, Stolley and colleagues (Stolley, Becker, Lasagna, McEvilla, & Sloane, 1972) concluded from in-depth interviews with primary care physicians about prescribing practices that younger physicians—more recent graduates who had taken additional courses and received postgraduate training, and with several years' experience in practice—were more appropriate in their drug prescribing than older physicians. Also, physicians who were concerned with both psychosocial and quality dimensions of medical care, as compared with others, were better and more appropriate drug prescribers (Stolley et al., 1972).

Earlier in the book (Chapters 3 and 4), we discussed variation in practices based on doctors' and patients' sociodemographic characteristics. Here we will comment on how sociodemographic variables may relate to quality of care.

There is some evidence that there are small but consistent differences in the cognitive and humanistic skills of male and female physicians entering internal medicine. A study by Day and associates (Day, Norcini, Shea, & Benson, 1989) compared program directors' ratings of overall clinical competence and its specific components and pass rates for the 14,340 men and women taking the American Board of Internal Medicine (ABIM) certifying examinations in internal medicine in 1984–87. Directors of residency training programs routinely rate several aspects of the competence of residents at the time of their application for admission to the ABIM Exam. These ratings are based on long-standing observation of the resident's performance throughout the residency training. Often, the director will solicit additional input from others who have worked with the resident and who may comment on his or her clinical performance. Finally, these ratings also provide information on the noncognitive aspects of competence that may not be captured on a written test, such as humanism.

The average program directors' ratings of overall competence were slightly higher for men than women. The greatest differences in ratings of specific components of competence were in the areas of medical knowledge and procedural skills, where men were rated higher than women. However, in terms of humanistic qualities, women were rated higher than men. Consistent with program directors' ratings, scores on the certifying examination reflected slightly better performance for men than women regardless of the type of residency or quality of medical school attended.

What research there is on male and female doctors' technical performance once in full-time practice suggests little difference between the sexes. Palmer's study of doctors in Boston is the most comprehensive study of male and female technical performance (Hall, Palmer, Orav, Hargraves, Wright, & Louis, 1990). Mostly, male and female doctors did not differ. However, female doctors scored much higher on the frequency with which they checked for breast and cervical cancer in women. When dealing with medical tasks uniquely relevant to their own sex, these women doctors may have experienced a heightened identification or empathy that led them to be more thorough.

The patient's sex also had effects in this study. Doctors (whether male or female) treated young girls with urinary tract infections more thoroughly than they treated young boys, but the exact opposite occurred for ear infection— there, boys got better treatment. This apparent inconsistency makes sense if one takes into account which sex is more prone to these conditions. Girls are more prone to urinary infections, boys to earaches. It appears, then, that doctors are likely to follow accepted procedure best when treating the sex that is "known" for the condition. Most likely this happens because the doctor expects to find certain conditions in a male (or female) patient and is more prepared to deal with them when they are found. Of course this makes no rational sense. A girl with an ear infection will suffer the same complications and possible permanent damage as a boy if the condition is not treated properly.

If this hypothesis about doctor expectations is correct, we should find the same pattern for other medical conditions associated mainly with one sex. For heart disease we do. Among men and women with the same extent of symptoms, women receive coronary angiography (a key diagnostic test) far less frequently than men do (Tobin, Wassertheil-Smoller, Wexler, Steingart, Budner, Lense, & Wachspress, 1987).

Other physician demographics have also been looked at in research on performance quality. Such factors include whether doctors were board certified, whether they went to medical school in the United States, and whether they took continuing education courses. These kinds of background traits have usually been weak or conflicting predictors of quality (Palmer & Reilly, 1979).

VARIATION IN QUALITY OF CARE AND HEALTH CARE SETTING

Although doctors and patients are the key actors as far as the medical visit is concerned, that visit takes place within the larger context of the organization of care. Interest in organizational influences on medical care has grown greatly now that health care is provided in many settings and with many payment mechanisms. The traditional fee-for-service model, whereby patients pay individual practitioners per visit or per episode, is dwindling. Now there are many insurance plans and reimbursement systems (for example, for determining how much hospitals are reimbursed for the care of an elderly patient). A major event in American health care has been the astonishing growth of the health maintenance organization, or HMO.

Each plan, scheme, and form of organization has implications for the kind and quality of care received by patients. For example, the federal government's policy of paying hospitals according to a Medicare patient's diagnosis, and not according to his or her actual medical expenses, is believed to result in patients being discharged "quicker and sicker." As another example, prepayment, the defining feature of the HMO, promotes comprehensive health care but also creates disincentives for the HMO to provide expensive services.

Even the length of the visit, which one would like to think depends on the gravity of the condition, or at least on the practice style of the doctor, is often, in fact, determined by the scheduling practices of whatever clinic or setting one goes to. This aspect of bureaucratization makes doctors in HMOs especially unhappy. Since more and more health care is delivered in such "managed care" settings, it will be important to follow the course of doctors' job satisfaction, for doctors' job satisfaction is correlated with how satisfied their patients are (Linn, Brook, Clark, Davies, Fink, & Kosecoff, 1985). Whether this is because organizational features have a common impact on both doctor and patient, or because dissatisfied doctors pass their dissatisfaction along to their patients by the manner of treatment (or vice versa), is not yet known.

Research on inpatient care has found that when a hospital is larger, nonprofit, and affiliated with a medical school for teaching and research, it tends to deliver higher-quality care. Care is also enhanced when the consequences of care are more visible, as when there are more frequent reports of medical staff activities or efforts to acquaint the medical staff with the quality of their past performance (Palmer, Louis, Hsu, Peterson, Rothrock, Strain, Thompson, & Wright, 1985; Rhee, 1983). Hospitals also differ widely in how often their patients die during their stay, even after taking into account the fact that some hospitals serve sicker people than others. A close look reveals at least part of the explanation: the more experienced the hospital is in performing similar types of operations, the better are one's chances of getting out alive (Kelly & Hellinger, 1986).

In fact, the kind of hospital in which physicians practice has more impact on the quality of care delivered than factors related to an individual doctor's training and experience (Rhee, 1977). The relative importance of physician versus hospital factors to quality of care was explored in a study of 454 physicians and 2,517 of their patients discharged from 22 hospitals in the state of Hawaii. Physician behavior for each patient discharge was examined in light of medical norms for each of 15 diagnostic categories created by expert panels to determine quality of care ratings.

The authors found that while the level of physician training was generally equal across hospitals, the site of care was associated with a tremendous performance difference—large teaching hospitals offered better care than community hospitals. Where a physician worked had a greater influence on the quality of performance than did personal factors that presumably reflect knowledge and skills, such as type of medical school attended, time in practice, and degree of specialization. There was some mutual influence of these factors, however. The kind of hospital was less important for highly trained physicians; well-trained physicians did better than poorly trained physicians in any setting. However, poorly trained physicians did much better when they worked at a teaching hospital than when they were associated with a community hospital (Rhee, 1977).

To summarize, medical care is not always good, and it is extremely variable. Much of this variability we believe to result from deficiencies in the talk between doctors and patients, and some of it, no doubt, is exacerbated by the system of care within which the care is delivered.

MEDICAL SCHOOL TRAINING AND QUALITY OF CARE

Some seeds of the quality of care problem are planted early in the medical education process, in the very midst of everyone's highest aspirations for the doctors of the future. This irony stems from a prevailing value system rooted both in academic medicine and high technology.

Students get insufficient opportunity to interact with patients and therefore to acquire interviewing skills. Further, what experience they have with patients tends mainly to be with those who have already been admitted to the hospital. These patients are usually quite sick, and there is an inevitable (and often justifiable) neglect of learning a range of skills appropriate to relating to the whole person, in favor of perfecting a much smaller repertoire of life-sustaining, or highly focused, disease-specific, medical actions.

The emphasis on learning at the bedside has other implications too. Students may not only lack experience with routine cases, but, worse, some undoubtedly learn to devalue routine cases; they learn to expect routine cases to provide little reward and challenge. Of course, such cases may be short on medical complexity in the strict sense, but are long on issues of compliance, lifestyle, emotional distress, and coping—issues that are plenty challenging, but are outside the narrow bounds of medicine as it is defined, for the most part, in medical school.

Academic medicine places high value not only on "real" medical problems but also on difficult ones—partly because of the drama, partly because of the respect gained when one is able to solve a diagnostic riddle or make correct judgments under pressure. We suspect there are many physicians in practice today who would be extremely unlikely to make an error on a serious or complex case but who are casual about following accepted good procedure on routine conditions such as urinary tract infection, ear infection, and follow-up of a low blood count, simply because these cases appear easy and uninteresting. But these cases are the stuff of most doctor visits. Errors on these easy conditions can have serious clinical ramifications, and further-more, even minor errors accumulate over millions of office visits to produce higher average costs of care and much accumulated discomfort and incon-venience for the patients involved.

Another feature of medical education that has long been talked of as a factor in quality of patient care is the extreme overwork demanded of interns and residents. As described earlier in detail (Chapter 4), it is not uncommon for interns and residents to work eighty or even one hundred hours a week (Mizrahi, 1986). Ironically, pride in working while totally exhausted, and even sick, is deeply ingrained in physicians during their early training. Perri Klass, a Boston pediatrician, describes the training atmosphere as "macho," demanding perseverance through fatigue and illness: "Interns don't stay home unless they're hospitalized or dead" (Klass, 1987).

This of course means these young physicians are treating patients who are critically ill when they themselves are in a state of exhaustion. This is despite commonsense knowledge that mistakes are made, judgment clouded, and perhaps quality of care jeopardized under these circumstances. An investigation of resident and intern mistakes was undertaken by Wu and associates (Wu, Folkman, McPhee, & Lo, 1991). A survey was mailed to residents and interns in three large internal medicine training programs associated with medical schools and academic hospitals. Questionnaires were filled out anonymously to assure confidentiality. Approximately 45% of those surveyed responded to the questionnaire and reported a mistake that they had made during their training years.

Among the most frequently reported mistakes were missed diagnosis, errors in prescribing and dosing of drugs, and faulty communication. For instance, one resident missed an intern's dosing error—an 80-milligram dose of cardiac medication was transcribed as 180 milligrams. The patient was found dead two hours after the first dose. An example of faulty communication was noted wherein a resident accepted misinformation from the emergency department physician that a patient being admitted was not to be resuscitated, a "no code." Subsequently, the resident found out from the patient's family and personal physician that the patient was not a "no code," but by that point the patient had not been treated aggressively, and died twenty-four hours later.

The causes of the mistakes were varied and were often attributed to more than one precipitating factor. Inexperience was cited more frequently than any other cause, including an insufficient knowledge base, insufficient experience, and a failure to ask for advice. Job overload was also frequently cited as a leading cause of mistakes—respondents noted that they had "too many other tasks" and were fatigued when the mistake occurred. Faulty judgment in complex cases, hesitation, and indecision were also noted.

The consequences of these mistakes were very serious. Ninety percent of the residents reported that the patient suffered a significant adverse effect, including prolonged hospital stay or death. Despite the consequences of the mistakes, physicians discussed them with patients in only 24% of cases. The mistakes were discussed with supervisors in 54% of cases, and other physicians in 88%; 5% of the physicians did not tell anyone about the mistake. The authors note that disclosure of a mistake may foster learning by compelling the physician to take responsibility for it and to get through the guilt and avoidance that the experience is likely to produce.

The overwork of house staff is sometimes defended as an important feature of medical training, as an efficient way of exposing house staff to a high volume of highly varied cases, and as an optimal way to teach doctors quick, automatic judgment (if you can do the right thing when you are asleep, then you have really learned your business). However, issues of medical malpractice have been raised by the lay press with concerns that overworked and sleep-deprived residents may be more prone to make serious and sometimes deadly mistakes (Asch & Parker, 1988). Commentators in this area feel that this change is imminent as it becomes increasingly clear to society that the current process of training of physicians is dangerous to both the trainees and their patients (Colford & McPhee, 1989).

Fatigue among interns and residents is an especially visible source of variations in care, but other aspects of training have also been studied in relation to quality. Grades in medical school are generally not markers of future performance quality, and when evidence suggests such a relationship, it is probably due to the fact that better medical students continue for longer training (i.e., enter specialties), and longer training is associated with quality (Palmer & Reilly, 1979). However, a qualification to this finding is that even physicians who have continued in training and have joined specialties still give less than optimal care when they practice outside their area of specialty. This has been shown, for example, when surgeons treat nonsurgical cases and when psychiatrists are made responsible for general medical or surgical care (Palmer & Reilly, 1979). Thus, having not only more training but also the right training matters greatly in the quality of care.

Although grades in medical school are generally weak predictors of later performance, tests of medical knowledge have been shown to be more strongly related to performance. In our study of primary care physicians in Pennsylvania, a paper-and-pencil test of their knowledge of lung disease was a strong predictor of the quality of their actual performance with live (but simulated) patients two full years later (Hall & Roter, 1988). Those who knew the most on the test were the ones who received the highest scores on clinical expertise in the later office visits. They also provided the most medical information to the patients, but spent much less time in nonmedical small talk than did doctors who had not scored as well on the paper-and-pencil test. Thus, the knowledgeable doctors—two years later—were superior in both clinical medicine and the communication of information, while some of the less knowledgeable ones may have tried to mask their shortcomings with camaraderie.

Perhaps it is not surprising that a doctor's knowledge of medicine should be related to actual "doctoring" with patients, but in fact this issue has been looked at rather infrequently. And although we can assume that good knowledge of textbook medicine must underlie good practice, good practice involves much else, only some of which is emphasized (or even taught at all) in medical school.

REFERENCES

Asch, D., & Parker, R. (1988). The Libby Zion case. *New England Journal of Medicine, 318,* 771–774.

Bensing, J. (1991). *Doctor-patient communication and the quality of care: An observation study into affective and instrumental behavior in general practice.* Utrecht, Netherlands: NIVEL.

Colford, J. M., & McPhee, S. J. (1989). The ravelled sleeve of care: Managing the stresses of residency training. *Journal of the American Medical Association, 261,* 889–893.

Day, S.C., Norcini, J. J., Shea, J. A., & Benson, J. A., Jr. (1989). Gender differences in the clinical competence of residents in internal medicine. *Journal of General Internal Medicine, 4,* 309–312.

Domenighetti, G., Luraschi, P., Casabianca, A., Gutzwiller, F., Spinelli, A., Pedrinis, E., & Repetto, F. (1988). Effect of information campaign by the mass media on hysterectomy rates. *The Lancet,* 24–31 December, 1470–1473.

Epstein, A. M., Begg, C. B., & McNeil, B. J. (1986). The use of ambulatory testing in prepaid and fee-for-service group practices: Relation to perceived profitability. *New England Journal of Medicine, 314,* 1089–1094.

Epstein, A. M., & McNeil, B. J. (1987). Variations in ambulatory test use: What do they mean? *Medical Clinics of North America, 71,* 705–717.

Hall, J. A., Epstein, A. M., & McNeil, B. J. (1989). Multidimensionality of health status in an elderly population: Construct validity of a measurement battery. *Medical Care, 27,* S168–S177.

Hall, J. A., Palmer, R. H., Orav, E. J., Hargraves, J. L., Wright, E. A., & Louis, T. A. (1990). Performance, quality, gender and professional role: A study of physicians and nonphysicians in sixteen ambulatory care practices. *Medical Care, 28,* 489–501.

Hall, J. A., & Roter, D. L. (1988). Physicians' knowledge and self-reported compliance promotion as predictors of performance with simulated lung disease patients. *Evaluation and the Health Professions, 11,* 306–317.

Hall, J. A., Roter, D. L., & Katz, N. R. (1987). Task versus socioemotional behaviors in physicians. *Medical Care, 25,* 399–412.

Hemminki, E. (1975). Review of literature on the factors affecting drug prescribing. *Social Science & Medicine, 9,* 111–115.

Kelly, J. V., & Hellinger, F. J. (1986). Physician and hospital factors associated with mortality of surgical patients. *Medical Care, 24,* 785–800.

Klass, P. (1987). *A not entirely benign procedure: Four years as a medical student.* New York: Signet.

Linn, L. S., Brook, R. H., Clark, V. A., Davies, A. R., Fink, A., & Kosecoff, J. (1985). Physician and patient satisfaction as factors related to the organization of internal medicine group practices. *Medical Care, 23,* 1171–1178.

Mishler, E. G. (1984). *The discourse of medicine: Dialectics of medical interviews.* Norwood, N.J.: Ablex.

Mizrahi, T. (1986). *Getting rid of patients: Contradictions in the socialization of physicians.* New Brunswick, N.J.: Rutgers University Press.

Palmer, R. H., Louis, T. A., Hsu, L-N., Peterson, H. F., Rothrock, J. K., Strain, R., Thompson, M. S., & Wright, E. A. (1985). A randomized controlled trial of quality assurance in sixteen ambulatory care practices. *Medical Care*, *23*, 751–770.

Palmer, R. H., & Reilly, M. C. (1979). Individual and institutional variables which may serve as indicators of quality of medical care. *Medical Care*, *17*, 693–717.

Palmer, R. H., Strain, R., Maurer, J.V.W., Rothrock, J. K., & Thompson, M. S. (1984). Quality assurance in eight adult medicine group practices. *Medical Care*, *22*, 632–643.

Palmer, R. H., Strain, R., Maurer, J.V.W., & Thompson, M. S. (1984). A method for evaluating performance of ambulatory pediatric tasks. *Pediatrics*, *73*, 269–277.

Rhee, S. (1977). Relative importance of physicians' personal and situational characteristics for the quality of patient care. *Journal of Health and Social Behavior*, *18*, 10–15.

Rhee, S. O. (1983). Organizational determinants of medical care quality: A review of the literature. In Luke, R. D., Krueger, J. C., & Modrow, R. E. (Eds.), *Organization and change in health care quality assurance*. Rockville, Md.: Aspen.

Roter, D. L., & Hall, J. A. (1987). Physicians' interviewing styles and medical information obtained from patients. *Journal of General Internal Medicine*, *2*, 325–329.

Roter, D. L., Hall, J. A., & Katz, N. R. (1987). Relations between physicians' behaviors and analogue patients' satisfaction, recall, and impressions. *Medical Care*, *25*, 437–451.

Sanazaro, P. J., & Worth, R. M. (1985). Measuring clinical performance of individual internists in office and hospital practice. *Medical Care*, *23*, 1097–1114.

Stolley, P. D., Becker, M. H., Lasagna, L., McEvilla, J. D., & Sloane, L. M. (1972). The relationship between physician characteristics and prescribing appropriateness. *Medical Care*, *10*, 17–28.

Tobin, J. N., Wassertheil-Smoller, S., Wexler, J. P., Steingart, R. M., Budner, N., Lense, L., & Wachspress, J. (1987). Sex bias in considering coronary bypass surgery. *Annals of Internal Medicine*, *107*, 19–25.

Wang, V., Terry, P., Flynn, B., Williamson, J., Green, L., & Faden, R. (1979). Evaluation of continuing medical education for chronic obstructive pulmonary diseases. *Journal of Medical Education*, *54*, 803–811.

Wu, A. W., Folkman, S., McPhee, S. J., & Lo, B. (1991). Do house officers learn from their mistakes? *Journal of the American Medical Association*, *265*, 2089–2094.

8

Consequences of Talk: The Relationship of Talk to Patient Outcomes

To study the process of medical care, one focuses primarily on the physician. But the patient becomes the center of attention when one turns to the consequences of that care. The patient perspective has been investigated in terms of perception—how satisfied the patient is with care received; it has been investigated in terms of patient behavior—how likely the patient is to comply with therapeutic regimens; and, finally, in terms of effect—how much better the patient is as a result of care.

Predominantly, communication researchers interested in patient consequences have studied the first two outcomes: patient satisfaction with care and compliance with doctors' recommendations. Dissatisfied patients are less likely to return for visits and more likely to switch doctors and health plans. Dissatisfaction, because it implies low trust, also surely undermines the nonspecific healing mechanisms implied in placebo and suggestion effects. And a dissatisfied patient almost by definition will miss out on the rapport and reassurance that is part of a good doctor-patient relationship. Satisfaction is also linked with patient compliance—more satisfied patients are more likely to follow medical recommendations.

Medical recommendations run the gamut from taking a single pill or following a complex drug regimen, to seeking preventive care and returning for follow-up appointments, to modifying aspects of one's lifestyle. Noncompliance with recommendations jeopardizes patients' health and well-being, interferes with the doctor's therapeutic efforts, and leads to wasted health resources (DiMatteo & DiNicola, 1982). Failure to follow drug regimens adequately, for instance, has been linked to diminished therapeutic effect for at least half of patients for whom drugs are prescribed (Haynes, 1976).

While satisfaction and compliance issues have dominated the research, there is a small and extremely important body of work that has investigated the consequences of doctor-patient communication on measures of health status (Kaplan, Greenfield, & Ware, 1989). Included among these measures are actual physiologic indicators. For instance, an appropriate indicator for diabetic patients is blood sugar monitored through levels of glycosylated hemoglobin ($HbA1_c$), and for hypertensive patients it is blood pressure. In addition, such measures as functional status (the patient's ability to perform usual daily routines) and a patient's overall sense of well-being are important indicators of how well a patient is doing.

This chapter will explore the body of research that links patient satisfaction, compliance, and several health status measures to doctor-patient communication.

PATIENT SATISFACTION

Although studied often, patients and their points of view in terms of satisfaction with care have not always been highly regarded by the medical profession and by researchers. Patients have been disparaged on account of their supposed ignorance of proper medicine, their tendency to be taken in by charlatans with good bedside manners, and their distorted views of what is important in medical care. Distortion is, of course, in the eye of the beholder. As patienthood takes on more consumerist qualities, and the medical system becomes more competitive, health care will cater more to what its managers believe patients want. The question, however, is what do patients want?

Perhaps the most common misgiving of the medical profession in regard to patients' evaluations of care is that they are thought to be unable to distinguish good from poor technical care—that is, the skills of diagnosis and treatment. We cannot say definitely how true or untrue this assumption is, for only recently did researchers even ask the question. Nevertheless, recent studies do suggest that patients are sensitive to variations in quality and are more satisfied when quality is high.

An example is a study of patients who came to an emergency room for treatment of burns (Linn, 1982). Physicians' technical performance was measured by researchers who scored the medical record for whether or not appropriate actions were taken. When the physicians performed better in these strictly medical tasks, their patients were more satisfied than when they performed worse. Although this study suggests that patients recognize good care when they see it, no one yet knows the limits of patients' ability to make such discriminations (and there certainly are limits, for no one could expect a lay person to understand many of the fine points of medical science).

Research has definitely shown that patients have reasonably accurate perceptions of the interpersonal manner of the physician and can report the extent and nature of communication received from the physician. Moreover, patient satisfaction studies have reflected patients' abilities to recognize variations in medical care. In these studies, patients are not always asked directly about their satisfaction. Sometimes they are asked merely to describe their care, and the investigator infers from the answer how satisfied they are. For example, agreement with the statement "My doctor answered all my questions fully" would be assumed to indicate high satisfaction because it is assumed a patient would want this to happen.

Table 8.1 shows characteristic items that might be used to measure a patient's satisfaction. These are arranged, from top to bottom, to reflect the relative frequency with which these different aspects of medical care are asked about in research. Most often, patients are asked about their satisfaction with the humaneness or interpersonal qualities of their doctor, and least often about their satisfaction with the attention given to personal (not medical) problems or problems of living (Hall & Dornan, 1988a).

Patients are generally rather satisfied with the doctor overall, and with the doctor's humaneness, technical competence, and outcome of care. These elements received the highest patient ratings (ranks one through four respectively) out of eleven satisfaction elements in over 107 published studies (Hall & Dornan, 1988a). Intermediate rankings, five through seven, were given to facilities, continuity of care, and access to care, respectively. The lowest ranks, eight through eleven, were found in regard to physicians' informativeness, medical care cost, bureaucracy, including how long one waits at the doctor's office, and, finally, physicians' attention to psychosocial problems.

The relative satisfaction rankings may reflect actual performance of the medical system, wherein some aspects of care may be emphasized over others—for example, technical skills over psychological support. Seen in this light, greater relative satisfaction with technical quality could mean that the health care systems emphasize technical performance to the relative neglect of patient needs that fall outside of a biomedical definition of health. These would include intellectual needs to be informed, psychological needs to be reassured and seen in the context of both social and biomedical problems, and economic needs for affordable health care and the avoidance of long waiting times (Hall & Dornan, 1988a).

The questions in Table 8.1 might be useful for readers to think about during, and after, a visit to a doctor. They might also be useful for a practitioner to think about in trying to take the patient's perspective in the visit. The exercise of thinking systematically about what the doctor does and

Table 8.1
Patients' Satisfaction with Medical Care: Sample Items

Item	Aspect of Medical Care
How satisfied are you with . . .	
. . . the respect accorded you by your doctor?	Humaneness
. . . how carefully your doctor listened to what you had to say?	
. . . the explanations given you by the doctor?	Informativeness
. . . the answers you got to your questions?	
. . . the doctor's performance overall?	Quality
. . . the quality of care you received today?	
. . . the health maintenance organization you belong to?	Overall
. . . your stay in the hospital?	
. . . the expertise of your doctor?	Technical
. . . how thoroughly your doctor examined you?	Competence
. . . how long you waited in the waiting room before seeing the doctor?	Bureaucracy
. . . the way the receptionist treated you?	
. . . how long it takes you to get an appointment?	Access to Care
. . . how far from your home your doctor's office is?	
. . . your ability to pay for good medical care?	Cost
. . . the amount charged by your doctor for a visit?	
. . . the appearance of the clinic?	Facilities
. . . how modern the equipment is?	
. . . the pain relief you experienced?	Outcome
. . . the resolution of your medical problem?	
. . . your ability to see the same doctor each time you need one?	Continuity
. . . the continuity of care you receive at this clinic?	
. . . how much attention the doctor paid to problems at home or at work?	Address of Psychosocial
. . . how much the doctor let you tell about any anxiety or depression you've had lately?	Problems

Note: These questions might be answered on a rating scale that goes from 1 to 6, where 1=very dissatisfied, 2=moderately dissatisfied, 3=slightly dissatisfied, 4=slightly satisfied, 5=moderately satisfied, and 6=very satisfied.

does not do, and how one reacts to it, tells a great deal not only about the doctor but about one's own expectations and values. This exercise can be especially useful for those who pay repeated visits to the same doctor or facility, since ratings can be compared between visits.

Although in Table 8.1 all the questions refer to one's own doctor or recent experiences, sometimes the questions used in research refer to doctors or medical care in general. This difference produces revealing results. To demonstrate this, readers could consider how they would respond to the following:

1. My doctor inspires a great deal of confidence in me.

    Agree strongly

    Agree moderately

    Agree weakly

    Disagree weakly

    Disagree moderately

    Disagree strongly

2. My doctor always treats me with utmost respect. (Answer these and the remainder using the same six options.)
3. My doctor often fails to provide information on my medical condition.

Now, compare your answers to the following:

4. Doctors inspire a great deal of confidence in me.
5. Doctors always treat their patients with utmost respect.
6. Doctors often fail to provide information on a patient's medical condition.

Most people score as more satisfied when describing their personal care than when describing care in general. If one thinks a moment, the illogic of this pattern of results becomes apparent. It is, of course, impossible for everyone's own care to be better than what is generally available. People display this same bias or illusion when rating many other facets of life. For example, people believe they are more happily married than average, and although women acknowledge that sex discrimination is common, most stoutly maintain that they are not discriminated against in their careers.

People do have strong needs to maintain their positive self-image and a sense of personal control. Perhaps they exaggerate the positive quality of their own medical experiences in order to maintain this sense of self-worth. The need to look good to oneself may be particularly strong when the issue in question involves choice, such as when one has chosen one's doctor or setting of health care.

Audiotapes and other objective records of doctor-patient interaction, which tell about events in the medical visit itself, can be used in conjunction with satisfaction data to explore factors associated with higher and lower satisfaction. Studies of this kind reveal that the social climate established in the visit appears to be a major determinant of satisfaction. Satisfaction is increased when physicians treat patients in a more partnerlike manner: when more positively toned words are spoken, such as statements of agreement; when fewer negative words are spoken, such as criticism; when more social conversation occurs, such as greetings and nonmedical chit-chat; and when the physician treats the patient in a warmer and more immediate nonverbal manner, such as sitting closer or engaging in more eye contact (Hall, Roter, & Katz, 1988). All of these behaviors suggest the way people act when they like someone. Indeed, research shows that when doctors like their patients, their patients are more satisfied with them (Hall, Epstein, DeCiantis, & McNeil, 1993; Like & Zyzanski, 1987).

In addition to specific behaviors, styles of communication have been related to patient satisfaction. The patient-centered interviewing style, in which the patient's point of view is actively sought and input facilitated through open expression of concerns and question asking, is positively associated with patient satisfaction (Stewart, 1984). In a similar vein, Buller and Buller (1985) found that an affiliative style, composed of communication behaviors designed to establish and maintain a positive relationship between physician and patient, such as friendliness, interest, empathy, a nonjudgmental attitude, and a social orientation, predicted patient satisfaction to a much greater degree than a more dominant communication style.

An interviewing style that focuses on psychosocial concerns is also related to patient satisfaction (Bertakis, Roter, & Putnam, 1991). We found that while physician question asking about biomedical topics was negatively related to patient satisfaction, question asking about psychosocial topics was positively related. Also, physician counseling for psychosocial issues and patient talk to the physician in the psychosocial domain were positively related to patient satisfaction.

The emotional climate is not the only factor that predicts satisfaction. The strongest predictor among variables measured during the medical visit is how much information is given to the patient. Such information could be on diagnosis, the causes and course of a disease, or on possible treatments and what they entail. Patients who get more information are more satisfied than patients who get less (Hall, Roter, & Katz, 1988). This speaks to the high value placed on information by patients. The correlation of information to satisfaction could reflect not only a patient's desire for information per se; it could also indicate how patients feel about doctors who give more information. Patients may reason that a doctor who bothers to give more information is nicer or more concerned about them as people. Thus, two values may operate simultaneously—the value placed by patients on medical information, and the value placed on having a humane and involved physician.

The physician's technical competence as demonstrated in the visit is also reflected in a patient's satisfaction. Linn (1982), in the study mentioned earlier, scored competence on the basis of what was written in medical charts. Studies that use audiotapes also score competence, but differently, by applying agreed-on standards of good medical care to what was said by the doctors during the visit, as well as what was done. So, for example, certain questions ought to be asked of a patient with chest pains. Studies of this type also show that patients are more satisfied when the physician is more competent according to these technical standards (Hall & Roter, 1988).

We know that there are differences in the behavior of medical residents versus more experienced physicians. The younger doctors have been shown to behave more competently, both technically and interpersonally, to engage in more nonmedical talk, and to conduct longer visits (Roter, Hall, & Katz, 1988). Other research shows that patients like it when their doctors have these traits. It is therefore not surprising to learn that patients are more satisfied, on average, with residents than with more experienced doctors (Hall & Dornan, 1988b).

Another doctor trait associated with satisfaction is nonverbal communication skill. Several studies have been conducted exploring the ways in which emotions and feelings may be transmitted during the medical visit. It was found that doctors' feelings toward patients, reflected in how they talked about patients, was very much related to how they actually talked to patients. Physicians who feel critical and rejecting toward particular patients convey these feelings through their tone of voice. The doctor who speaks about patients in a coldly autocratic way tends also to speak to them in the same manner; physicians who speak about patients in a warm and caring way tend to speak to them in a warm and honest tone of voice (Rosenthal, Vannicelli, & Blanck, 1984).

Nonverbal skill has also been extensively studied by DiMatteo and her colleagues at the University of California (DiMatteo, Hays, & Prince, 1986). As described in Chapter 4, DiMatteo tests doctors' abilities in nonverbal communication using standardized testing situations. One test measures how accurately they can recognize emotions in people's faces and voices; another measures how accurately they can express themselves emotionally through facial expression and voice tone. Having measured these skills in doctors, DiMatteo then asks their patients about their satisfaction with the care provided.

This research has shown that the patients of doctors with more developed nonverbal communication skills are the most satisfied. Although DiMatteo has not yet studied the doctors she has tested in actual interaction with their patients, one can speculate on what the high- and low-scoring doctors do that influences patient satisfaction. We would guess that the more sensitive and expressive doctors interact with patients in a way that is more tuned in to the patients' needs. They may use their faces more effectively to communicate empathy, and they may be able to detect patients' feelings and thoughts that are not expressed through words. For example, a patient who hesitates to speak about a problem, who is nervous or frightened, or who is angry, may convey these feelings nonverbally in ways that only the more nonverbally sensitive physician can pick up. In order to produce higher satisfaction levels, however, these doctors would then have to act on their knowledge in ways that meet with patients' approval. They might be more likely to say, "You seem to have something else on your mind" to the hesitant patient, "I can see you are a bit worried about this test result" to the frightened one, or "I hope you'll let me know if I do anything you don't like" to the angry one.

Patients are also considerably more satisfied when continuity is greater— that is, when they see the same provider regularly rather than seeing a different face each time. We find this especially interesting not only because of what it suggests about patients' values, but also because greater continuity has implications for the nature of doctor-patient interaction. There is un- doubtedly more warmth and familiarity in more continuous relationships, with patients in such arrangements feeling that the doctor has a greater personal commitment to them. Whether the latter is true or not, patients probably reciprocate the sense of commitment by becoming more involved themselves, perhaps by taking a more active role, by better compliance with recommendations, or by feeling more confident of their right to speak and to ask questions freely.

Patients who are healthier are also more satisfied than those who are less healthy, whether health is defined in terms of physical disorders or emotional distress (Pascoe, 1983; Hall, Feldstein, Fretwell, Rowe, & Epstein, 1990). More than one explanation can be offered for this tendency. There is some evidence that dissatisfied patients may simply be dissatisfied people: patients who are dissatisfied with their medical care also tend to be dissatisfied with the government, the community, and other nonmedical aspects of their everyday life. Thus, to some extent their dissatisfaction with medical care may have nothing to do with the care per se but rather with their characteristic outlook.

But medical care could certainly play a part in the dissatisfaction of sicker and more emotionally distressed patients. For one thing, these patients interact more frequently with the medical care system, and therefore have many more opportunities to experience bad medicine or upsetting behavior on the part of health care providers. Those who experience more negative events because of more frequent trips to the doctor could certainly have lower satisfaction than those who visit less often.

Just this point has been demonstrated by a large survey of patients and doctors conducted in the early 1980s. The researchers found that patients who have suffered from a chronic condition for many years are more knowledgeable about what constitutes good medical practice for that condition and are more critical of the care they receive than are less experienced patients (Haug & Lavin, 1983).

Yet another explanation for the link between health and satisfaction may be that patients with more intractable problems experience less relief and therefore are likely to leave a doctor's office still feeling bad. Finally, and most pertinent to our interest in doctor-patient talk, is the possibility that doctors in general treat healthier patients differently than they treat less healthy ones. Doctors are uncomfortable around suffering, especially if they want to alleviate it but cannot. If a patient acts pathetic about how he or she feels physically, or breaks down and cries, a doctor may easily be unnerved at not knowing what to do or may get irritated if the schedule is disrupted. The net effect is that the sicker or more unhappy individual may receive more negative cues. Our recent research has indeed found that patients who were liked least by their doctors were also those with the worst physical and emotional health (Hall, Epstein, DeCiantis, & McNeil, 1993). Thus, the dissatisfaction of the sicker patient may stem in part from the behavior of doctors.

PATIENT COMPLIANCE

Prescriptions have become one of the predominant symbols of the medical visit, and this symbol appears meaningful to both doctors and patients. A common image depicted in pharmaceutical advertisements in medical journals is that of a physician's hand superimposed over the patient, symbolically protecting or encompassing the patient, suggesting that the drug be used as an extension of—if not a substitute for—the physician (Krantzler, 1986). Likewise, patients are bombarded with media images of the physician—both scientific and fatherly—linked to thousands of drug products. The role of drugs is central not only to the media image, but to the reality of medicine; two-thirds of medical visits result in a prescription being given (Rabin & Bush, 1975).

There is an irony here, however. It is clear that doctors very often write prescriptions; it is also clear that patients very often ignore them. Estimates of patient noncompliance rates with prescribed therapeutic regimens typically range from 30% to 60%, with most researchers agreeing that at least one-half of patients for whom drugs are prescribed fail to receive full benefit through inadequate adherence (Haynes, 1976). Yet doctors infrequently suspect that their patients are not taking their drugs exactly as prescribed. Patients rarely volunteer to their doctor that this may be the case, and doctors don't often ask.

Surely something is wrong. A particularly telling example concerns the mother of a fourteen-year-old girl diagnosed as having epilepsy during a hospitalization following a seizure. Medication was prescribed but was soon discontinued because there were no symptoms. The girl took no more medicine for five years, during which time she was apparently symptom-free. However, the girl's mother regularly went to her doctor to obtain repeat prescriptions, "in order to keep up the appearance of being a 'good' mother" (West, 1976, p. 29).

Prescription drugs are often overutilized, underutilized, or otherwise taken inappropriately. One study found that almost one-third of the patients who received prescriptions were using them in a manner that posed a serious threat to their health (Boyd, Covington, Stanaszek, & Coussons, 1974). While some portion of these errors is purposeful, as illustrated in the case above, it is likely that much of the problem can be attributed to poor instruction.

Again and again, the most important contribution to patient compliance with drug prescriptions appears to be the patient's understanding of the illness, the rationale and importance of the drug therapy, and the instructions for use. However, full discussion of these points in the medical visit is rare. Examining physicians' verbal instructions to patients during medical visits in which drugs were prescribed, Svarstad (1974) found no discussion at all for almost 20% of the drugs, and no information about the purpose and/or name of the drug in one-third of the cases. Advice on how long to take the drug was given in only 10% of the visits and how often to take the drug was mentioned in fewer than one out of five visits. These findings are not atypical; full and clear information about drugs is not very commonly given. A guide to full discussion of drugs is provided in Table 8.2.

We do know that when the doctor offers more information, more positive talk, and less negative talk, and asks fewer questions overall (but more questions about compliance in particular), the patient is more likely to be compliant (Hall, Roter, & Katz, 1988). Additionally, it was found that compliance was increased when providers took a more dominant role in the visit. The association of less question asking to more compliance is consistent with research that has found question asking to be inversely related to information giving (Hall, Roter, & Katz, 1987). Again, as mentioned earlier in this chapter, we believe that it is not only the substantive nature of the information given to patients that enhances patient compliance, but the

Table 8.2
Medication Checklist

>   The following points or issues should be discussed when any drugs are
>   prescribed.

1. Purpose and rationale for the medicine
2. Likely effect to be gained by taking the medicine and/or consequences of not taking the medicine
3. Name of the medicine
4. Amount of drug to be taken in a single dose
5. Total number of doses to be taken daily
6. Timing or sequence of doses
7. How the dose should be taken (with food, milk, etc.)
8. Maximum amount of the drug that can be used in one day (as with drugs to be taken as needed)
9. Length of time for which the medicine should be used
10. Other drugs, specific foods, or activities that should be avoided
11. Proper storage techniques
12. Possible or likely side effects

Also, questions about drugs prescribed in previous visits are important in order to check that regimens are being followed correctly, whether modifications are necessary, and whether any side effects have occurred.

attribution of caring and humaneness given by patients to an informative physician.

There is other evidence that emotion transmitted through the doctor's tone of voice has an important effect on the patient's likelihood of following the doctor's recommendations. For instance, hostility in physicians' tone of voice in speaking about alcoholic patients related to the failure of patients to go to an alcoholism treatment center (Milmoe, Rosenthal, Blane, Chafetz, & Wolf, 1967). Presumably, these doctors also displayed hostility and rejection in their tone of voice during medical visits, and patients responded by rejecting the doctors' suggestions for further treatment, even though that treatment was with other doctors in a different facility.

Our own research on physicians' voice tone similarly found a connection between the doctors' tone of voice and patients' subsequent behavior. We found that certain combinations of voice tone and actual words used by the doctor were related to patient satisfaction and keeping of appointments (Hall, Roter, & Rand, 1981). Other research found that physicians' sensitivity to expressed emotion was significantly related to their patients' behavior; the more sensitive physicians had fewer appointment cancellations that failed to be rescheduled (DiMatteo, Hays, & Prince, 1986). We believe the notion of reciprocity is operating in these studies. Physicians affect patients by their expressions, and this in turn influences such things as patients' feelings of satisfaction as well as actual behaviors, such as keeping appointments.

One might argue that emotional sensitivity is beyond conscious control, and that physicians should not be held accountable for such "emotional leaks," but the provision of verbal and written communication to patients is another matter.

Written instructions are not necessarily much more informative than verbal communication. In a review of pharmacy records covering some 2,000 prescriptions, researchers found that 15% had label instructions that read "PRN," indicating that the drug should be taken as needed, with no further guidance, while an additional 8% were labeled simply "as directed," with no additional directions (Covington, Porter, & See, 1979). It has been observed more than once that better instructions are provided for the proper utilization and maintenance of a new camera or automobile than to patients in regard to the drugs they receive.

It is also likely that other factors may be complicating drug communication. A specific diagnosis is made for only about half of the complaints brought to a doctor; however, drugs are often prescribed in these cases despite the absence of a diagnostic rationale and with the expectation of minimal effect, at best (Thomas, 1978). One can imagine that under these circumstances, doctors may not specify instructions to patients because they are not very confident that these drugs will in fact make much of a difference. Nonetheless, the drugs are prescribed, probably because the doctor thinks the patient wants them, rather than because they are clinically justified. And again, the notion of reciprocity may be operable. In light of the almost casual way in which most drugs are prescribed, the high rates of patient noncompliance might well be expected. There does not appear to be much relationship between patient compliance and the clinical justification for prescribing the drug; appropriate and effective drug regimens may be as poorly adhered to as drugs prescribed without a good clinical reason.

We certainly do not want to imply that all drugs are ineffective or act to the detriment of the patient. Clearly that is not true, but the issue of patient compliance with drug recommendations is a complex one, made more complex by a lack of communication and by inaccurately perceived expectations. One survey of doctors' prescribing habits found that most doctors estimate that four out of five of their patients expect a prescription at any given visit (Stimson & Webb, 1975). In fact, the expectation for a prescription may be built into a visit and reinforced by the doctor, rather than dictated by the patient. Since so many visits end with a prescription, it is reasonable for the patient to expect one. Ironically, the common belief among doctors that patients will be less satisfied with their visit and less likely to return for a follow-up visit if the doctor does not prescribe some medicine may be fostered by doctors themselves rather than by patients (Thomas, 1978).

In fact, patients may be more satisfied with their visits when they do not receive a prescription. Researchers in a large HMO found that patients who received a prescription as part of their medical visit had shorter visits, and were less satisfied with questions answered, interest shown, and explanations given by their physicians than were other patients (Wartman, Morlock, Malitz, & Palm, 1981). These findings suggest that prescriptions may be used by some doctors in lieu of good communication, and that this does not escape patients. One patient stated her feelings regarding what she saw as overeager prescribing by her doctor: "He's writing the name and address on the prescription while I'm talking to him. He doesn't know what I want, you know, I say 'One of these days—one of these days you'll write the prescription out before I even tell you what's wrong!' You know he's in the middle of doing it as I'm talking to him, you know" (Stimson, 1974, p. 102).

It is interesting to note how little discussion about the need or desire for a prescription actually takes place. Most patients are sensitive to doctors' feelings and do not want to appear to be rejecting an offer of help, even if they really would rather not have a prescription (Cartwright & Anderson, 1981). It is much easier to communicate a positive request rather than a negative one, particularly if this might be seen as a criticism of the doctor. As a result, doctors may be unaware when patients do not want drugs, but will generally know it when they do. Some doctors have adopted a policy of asking patients whether they want a prescription or not. The doctors report that they have been surprised at the numbers of patients who say they do not want one (Cartwright & Anderson, 1981).

These findings reflect a general trend among patients away from expectations for a prescription. In comparing the results of surveys taken in 1964 and 1977 in England, Cartwright found that the proportion of patients who said they had hoped for or expected a prescription or some medicine fell from 52% in 1966 to 41% in 1977. In 1977 patients were more critical of doctors for being inclined to give a prescription, whereas the opposite was true in the earlier survey. Shedding some light on the basis of this new attitude, the researchers found that patients often felt that they were given a prescription rather than a thorough examination, information, or discussion.

A second area in which patient cooperation with physician recommendations is apparently lacking is in relation to lifestyle change. Adherence to physicians' recommendations in regard to smoking, weight control, diet modification, exercise, and alcohol restriction is far less complete than drug compliance. These are, of course, difficult habits to change. Nonetheless, they are critical contributors to the chronic diseases, and responsibility to reduce these health-threatening habits is widely recognized as within the physician's purview.

Smoking in particular has been identified by the surgeon general as the single greatest cause of preventable death and disability in the United States; it is incontrovertibly linked to heart disease and stroke, as well as to a number of different types of cancer (U.S. Department of Health and Human Services, 1982). Physicians, well aware of the link between smoking and disease, believe that they have an obligation to counsel patients to quit smoking (Goldstein, Fischer, Richards, Goldstein, & Shank, 1987). Yet, only two-thirds of physicians surveyed report that they routinely advise their smoking patients to quit, and fewer than one-fourth offer any kind of systematic advice to their patients about quitting or refer them to outside sources of help for smoking cessation (Orleans, 1985).

This lack of active involvement by physicians in an area they readily acknowledge as extremely serious is attributed to a variety of factors, most notably a pessimism that doctors hold regarding their effectiveness in getting patients to quit smoking. Despite physicians' own reservations regarding their effectiveness, physician recommendations are indeed taken seriously by patients. A number of studies have shown that the single most important reason people give for quitting smoking is concern over their health, and that those who quit for health reasons or in response to physician advice are more likely to make repeated attempts to quit and are more likely to remain off cigarettes (Orleans, 1985).

The following statistics demonstrate that physicians are, in fact, more successful than they think they are: the national annual quit rate is 2% to 3%, whereas most studies in which physicians provide even minimal advice to patients show double and triple that rate. Typically, that is, 5% to 10% of patients so advised during the course of a routine visit can be expected to quit smoking. For the most part, this advice is given in a rather off-hand manner, taking a few minutes of time and without any consistent follow-up. When doctors make a special effort to counsel their patients to quit, particularly patients with some condition made worse by smoking, such as lung or heart disease, success in quitting is better than ten times the annual rate, from 30% to 50%.

The question of how much talk during the medical visit is actually devoted to issues of prevention has been addressed by Freeman (1987). Freeman noted that although the majority of physicians in her study said that they routinely talked about such health promotion issues as diet, exercise, drug and alcohol use, and family dynamics with their patients, this discussion was infrequent in the two hundred visits she observed. When health promotion issues were broached during the visit, they were almost always extremely short references that were quickly passed over. Moreover, doctors seemed most comfortable with lifestyle talk when it was directly tied to a specific medical condition, as when the doctor related diet and weight control to diabetes management, or smoking cessation to an episode of bronchitis.

Discussion was more awkward when health promotion talk was not tied to a specific condition, and in these instances, the discussion tended to occur toward the end of the visit. Doctors seemed somewhat embarrassed to be bringing up such topics as alcohol use or smoking and these comments sounded somehow off the record or not really as part of the business of the visit. Alternatively, the physician broached these subjects in a somewhat joking manner, perhaps anticipating patient rejection of prevention ideas. A recent Swedish study of lifestyle counseling in medical visits similarly found physicians uncomfortable with these tasks. While Swedish doctors more often introduced the topics of smoking and alcohol than their American counterparts, the discussion was equally characterized as awkward, shallow, and fragmentary (Larsson, Saljo, & Aronsson, 1987).

Our own analysis of lifestyle talk, however, produced somewhat different results (Russell & Roter, 1992). We analyzed audiotapes of interactions between 439 adult, chronic disease patients and 49 physicians in a variety of practice settings to explore the content, frequency, intensity, and dynamics of health promotion discussions during routine primary care medical visits. There was evidence of health promotion discussion in more than half of the audiotapes reviewed. Forty percent of the medical visits reflected some discussion about diet/weight control, at least twice the frequency of all other topics. Physical activity and stress were addressed in 20% and 17% of the visits, respectively. Discussion of cigarette smoking was less frequent than the preceding topics, averaging about 11%; cigarettes were discussed almost twice as often as the least common topic, alcohol consumption (6%).

In those visits in which lifestyle topics were discussed, the exchange lasted an average of four and a half minutes, or 20% of the total visit time. Nearly 60% of the discussions went beyond the perfunctory to attempts to counsel and/or encourage behavior change. To some extent, the difference between this report and others may be a function of changing times. As health promotion continues to gain prominence in both patient and physician consciousness, the changes in counseling frequency may reflect both greater patient demand for these services and greater physician comfort with promotion topics.

A patient's rejection of or inconsistent adherence to a doctor's recommendation is not a random occurrence. Surely all the responsibility for noncompliance cannot rest on the physician's shoulders; however, it is clear that in regard to drugs and lifestyle recommendations, in particular, messages are not conveyed in nearly as consistent and persuasive a manner as is desirable.

If physicians do not make the effort to convey fully the importance of the recommendations they make, and provide some guidance for the behaviors they advocate, patients cannot be expected to fulfill them faithfully. Again, our notion of reciprocity is relevant. Patients, we believe, will more fully comply with recommended behaviors when they believe that the doctor is serious about them. This message can be best conveyed to patients when physicians fully communicate their belief in the recommendations they make by taking the time to inform and counsel their patients.

PHYSIOLOGICAL OUTCOMES AND QUALITY OF LIFE CHANGES

It is one thing to argue that good doctor-patient communication leads to higher patient satisfaction and even compliance with recommendations, but quite another to link communication to specific health outcomes. However, this link has been established in both hospital and outpatient studies. Doctor-patient communication has been associated with improved recovery from surgery, decreased use of pain medication, and shortened hospital stays (Mumford, Schlesinger, & Glass, 1982), as well as physiological changes in blood pressure and blood sugar (Kaplan, Greenfield, & Ware, 1989).

The mechanism by which patients gain these health benefits is unclear; several alternatives are possible. First, as suggested earlier, a satisfied patient may have more confidence in his or her doctor, maximizing the nonspecific healing mechanism of the placebo effect. These patients may attribute more positive emotions to their doctors, viewing them as supportive, concerned, understanding, and reassuring. Furthermore, patients who faithfully follow through with medical recommendations maximize the therapeutic benefit from their regimens and make health care more effective.

But other mechanisms by which communication enhances patient health are also possible. Some kinds of communication may affect patients' health status by increasing self-confidence and motivation. Patients who perceive themselves as capable of affecting their own health in a positive manner may act healthier, and in fact become healthier, than those with poor self-concepts in terms of health and a lack of confidence in their own abilities. Moreover, an increased sense of participation in medical care decisions through more active, two-way communication may be linked with a positive perception of mastery and control over one's total environment, including health, leading to a more self-confident and powerful life outlook (Greenfield, Kaplan, Ware, Yano, & Frank, 1988).

Evidence of the link between communication and health comes from a wide literature, originating with a classic study in the area conducted by Egbert and associates (Egbert, Battit, Welch, & Bartlett, 1964). This study established an association between enhanced communication with hospital-ized patients and a variety of positive patient effects. In the controlled, randomized study, Egbert and his associates provided one group with special care consisting of a detailed discussion of postoperative pain, deep breathing, use of a trapeze, and other suggestions regarding comfortable movement after the operation. The special care group used about half the usual postoperative narcotics and were judged by their surgeons as ready for discharge from the hospital almost three days earlier than the control patients.

Far from unique, the findings from the Egbert study are consistent with a great number and variety of clinical reports (Mumford, Schlesinger, & Glass, 1982) in which the provision of information or psychological preparation to patients led to positive clinical outcomes. While these interventions and others will be described in greater detail in Chapter 9, our point here is that many studies have demonstrated that improved communication leads to positive patient outcomes.

A difficulty in the evaluation of the literature just mentioned, however, is that few of these studies actually observed exactly how the communication changes planned were actually put into effect. Fortunately, a handful of medical studies do exist in which a positive relationship between doctor and patient conversation and patient health status was found (Kaplan, Greenfield, & Ware, 1989).

Physiologic measures, particularly blood pressures, were found to im-prove in patients who were allowed uninterrupted expression of their health concerns by their doctors during office visits (Orth, Stiles, Scherwitz, Hennrikus, & Vallbona, 1987). The authors suggest that the relief to patients of unburdening to the provider might help relax them and consequently help reduce blood pressure.

A second study also found an association between doctor-patient talk and reduced blood pressure, as well as improvements in blood sugar control, perceived health status, and daily functioning. However, researchers found a different explanation of the mechanisms by which these health changes were accomplished (Kaplan, Greenfield, & Ware, 1989). In this study, more patient control, more engagement (marked especially by negative affect expressed by both patients and physicians), and more information provided by physicians during office visits were associated with better health status. The authors suggest that these aspects of communication reflect "healthy friction" or role tension between physicians and patients.

On the one hand, patients' assertions of control through more effective information seeking, and perhaps disagreements, transform an otherwise physician-dominated monologue into a two-way exchange in which the patient has an active role and an obvious stake. The patient thus engaged is invested, perhaps more than otherwise, in the process as well as the outcome of the visit. On the other hand, negative expressions of frustration by the physician with a patient who is not progressing as expected may be interpreted by the patient as an expression of caring on the part of the physician. In our own work, we have found that when physicians sound angry and anxious, their patients are more satisfied and compliant. We believe that they attribute more concern and sincerity to a physician who is emotionally engaged than to one who appears emotionally neutral (Hall, Roter, & Rand, 1981).

The talk of the medical visit has an influence on patients' health status over and above its specific contribution to diagnosis and therapeutic activities. We agree with Kaplan and associates that the physician-patient relationship is a primary bond that may act as a form of social support to influence patients' health status (Kaplan, Greenfield, & Ware, 1989).

REFERENCES

Bertakis, K. D. , Roter, D. , & Putnam, S. M. (1991). The relationship of physician medical interview style to patient satisfaction. *Journal of Family Practice*, *32*, 175–181.

Boyd, J. R., Covington, T. R., Stanaszek, W. F., & Coussons, R. T. (1974). Drug defaulting: Part I, Determinants of compliance. *American Journal of Hospital Pharmacy*, *31*, 362–366.

Buller, M. K., & Buller, D. B. (1985). Physicians' communication style and patient satisfaction. *Journal of Health and Social Behavior*, *28*, 375–388.

Cartwright, A., & Anderson, R. (1981). *General practice revisited: A second study of patients and their doctors*. London: Tavistock Publications.

Covington, T. R., Porter, M. E., & See, K. (1979). Improper prescription instructions: A factor in patient compliance. *Patient Counselling and Health Education*, *1*, 97–100.

DiMatteo, M. R., & DiNicola, D. D. (1982). *Achieving patient compliance*. New York: Pergamon Press.

DiMatteo, M. R., Hays, R. D., & Prince, L. M. (1986). Relationship of physicians' nonverbal communication skill to patient satisfaction, appointment non-compliance, and physician workload. *Health Psychology*, *5*, 581–594.

Egbert, L. D., Battit, G. E., Welch, C. E., & Bartlett, M. K. (1964). Reduction of postoperative pain by encouragement and instruction of patients. *New England Journal of Medicine*, *270*, 825–827.

Freeman, S. H. (1987). Health promotion talk in family practice encounters. *Social Science & Medicine*, *25*, 961-966.

Goldstein, S., Fischer, P. M., Richards, J. W., Goldstein, A., & Shank, J. C. (1987). Smoking counseling practices of recently trained family physicians. *Journal of Family Practice*, *24*, 195–197.

Greenfield, S., Kaplan, S. H., Ware, J. E., Jr., Yano, E. M., & Frank, H.J.L. (1988). Patients' participation in medical care: Effects on blood sugar control and quality of life in diabetes. *Journal of General Internal Medicine, 3*, 448–457.

Hall, J. A., & Dorman, M. C. (1988a). What patients like about their medical care and how often they are asked: A meta-analysis of the satisfaction literature. *Social Science & Medicine, 27*, 935–939.

Hall, J. A., & Dorman, M. C. (1988b). Meta-analysis of satisfaction with medical care: Description of research domain and analysis of overall satisfaction levels. *Social Science & Medicine, 27*, 637–644.

Hall, J. A., Epstein, A. M., DeCiantis, M. L., & McNeil, B. J. (1993). Physicians' liking for their patients: More evidence for the role of affect in medical care. *Health Psychology*, forthcoming.

Hall, J. A., Feldstein, M., Fretwell, M. D., Rowe, J. W., & Epstein, A. M. (1990). Older patients' health status and satisfaction with medical care in an HMO population. *Medical Care, 28*, 261–270.

Hall, J. A., & Roter, D. L. (1988). Physicians' knowledge and self-reported compliance promotion as predictors of performance with simulated lung disease patients. *Evaluation and the Health Professions, 11*, 306–317.

Hall, J. A., Roter, D. L., & Katz, N. R. (1987). Task versus socioemotional behaviors in physicians. *Medical Care, 25*, 399–412.

Hall, J. A., Roter, D. L., & Katz, N. R. (1988). Meta-analysis of correlates of provider behavior in medical encounters. *Medical Care, 26*, 657–675.

Hall, J. A., Roter, D. L., & Rand, C. S. (1981). Communication of affect between patient and physician. *Journal of Health and Social Behavior, 22*, 18–30.

Haug, M., & Lavin, B. (1983). *Consumerism in medicine: Challenging physician authority.* Beverly Hills, Calif.: Sage Publications.

Haynes, R. B. (1976). A critical review of the "determinants" of patient compliance with therapeutic regimens. In Sackett, D. L., & Haynes, R. B. (Eds.), *Compliance with therapeutic regimens.* Baltimore: Johns Hopkins University Press.

Kaplan, S. H., Greenfield, S., & Ware, J. E., Jr. (1989). Assessing the effects of physician-patient interactions on the outcomes of chronic disease. *Medical Care, 27*, S110–S127.

Krantzler, N. J. (1986). Media images of physicians and nurses in the United States. *Social Science & Medicine, 9*, 933–952.

Larsson, U. S., Saljo, R., & Aronsson, K. (1987). Patient-doctor communication on smoking and drinking: Lifestyle in medical consultations. *Social Science & Medicine, 25*, 1129–1137.

Like, R., & Zyzanski, S. J. (1987). Patient satisfaction and the clinical encounter: Social psychological determinants. *Social Science & Medicine, 24*, 351–357.

Linn, B. S. (1982). Burn patients' evaluation of emergency department care. *Annals of Emergency Medicine, 11*, 255–259.

Milmoe, S., Rosenthal, R., Blane, H. T., Chafetz, M. E., & Wolf, I. (1967). The doctor's voice: Postdictor of successful referral of alcoholic patients. *Journal of Abnormal Psychology, 72*, 78–84.

Mumford, E., Schlesinger, H. J., & Glass, G. V. (1982). The effects of psychologi-
    cal intervention on recovery from surgery and heart attacks: An analysis of
    the literature. *American Journal of Public Health, 72*, 141–151.

Orleans, C. T. (1985). Understanding and promoting smoking cessation: Overview
    and guidelines for physician intervention. *Annual Review of Medicine, 36*,
    51–61.

Orth, J. E., Stiles, W. B., Scherwitz, L., Hennrikus, D., & Vallbona, C. (1987).
    Patient exposition and provider explanation in routine interviews and hy-
    pertensive patients' blood pressure control. *Health Psychology, 6*(1), 29–
    42.

Pascoe, G. C. (1983). Patient satisfaction in primary health care: A literature review
    and analysis. *Evaluation and Program Planning, 6*, 185–210.

Rabin, D. L., & Bush, P. J. (1975). Who's using medicines? *Journal of Community
    Health, 1*, 106–117.

Rosenthal, R., Vannicelli, M., & Blanck, P. (1984). Speaking to and about patients:
    Predicting therapists' tone of voice. *Journal of Consulting and Clinical
    Psychology, 52*, 679–686.

Roter, D. L., Hall, J. A., & Katz, N. R. (1988). Physician-patient communication:
    A descriptive summary of the literature. *Patient Education and Counsel-
    ing, 12*, 99–119.

Russell, N. K., & Roter, D. L. (1992). Discussion of lifestyle topics with chronic
    disease patients in primary care medical visits. *American Journal of Public
    Health*, forthcoming.

Stewart, M. (1984). What is a successful doctor-patient interview? A study of
    interactions and outcomes. *Social Science & Medicine, 19*, 167–175.

Stimson, G. V. (1974). Obeying doctor's orders: A view from the other side. *Social
    Science & Medicine, 8*, 97–104.

Stimson, G. V., & Webb, B. (1975). *Going to see the doctor: The consultation
    process in general practice.* London: Routledge & Kegan Paul.

Svarstad, B. L. (1974). *The doctor-patient encounter: An observational study of
    communication and outcome.* Doctoral dissertation, University of Wiscon-
    sin, Madison.

Thomas, K. B. (1978). The consultation and the therapeutic illusion. *British Medi-
    cal Journal, 1*, 1327–1328.

U.S. Department of Health and Human Services. (1982). *The health consequences
    of smoking: Cancer.* Washington, D.C.: U.S. Government Printing Office.

Wartman, S. A., Morlock, L. L., Malitz, F. E., & Palm, E. (1981). Do prescriptions
    adversely affect doctor-patient interactions? *American Journal of Public
    Health, 71*, 1358–1361.

West, P. (1976). The physician and the management of childhood epilepsy. In
    Wadsworth, D. (Ed.), *Studies in everyday medical life.* Oxford: Martin
    Robertson.

9

Improving Talk through
Interventions

Imagine you are a man in your fifties, suffering a long two days in the hospital before your coronary bypass surgery. You have many questions about what's about to happen, and naturally you have fears too. Your hospital roommate is also awaiting surgery, but his is for fusing of the vertebrae in his back following a long history of disc trouble.

Suppose you are an eighty-year-old woman living in a nursing home. You can get around with your walker, but you often wonder what the point is—you seem to be losing some of your interest in things. One day the director, speaking to you and others from your floor, reminds you that you have responsibility for this as your home and should decide how you want your room to look.

Now, imagine you are a man of seventy-five, quite alert and energetic, but burdened with a growing list of ailments for which you regularly see your doctor. Sometimes you get confused about the increasingly complex explanations and drug regimens your doctor offers. In fact, the last time your daughter asked about your health, you found you didn't have the answers to several obviously important questions and had to admit you were not sure you were taking all the drugs you were supposed to.

How wonderful it would be if one could decrease the anxiety of the man in the hospital, increase the zest of the woman in the nursing home, and improve the elderly man's understanding of his regimen. Is it possible? And at what cost? How elaborate or intense an effort would have to be made by someone—doctors, social workers, psychologists—to achieve these gains? Has anyone tried?

Throughout this book, we have asserted our conviction that doctors and patients can change their interactions for the better, and we have spent most of these pages arguing that change is needed and theoretically possible. Now we intend to show that talk between doctors and patients (and, in one study, between patients) has been shown to be both cause and consequence of many important features of medical care.

We have been careful about using such terms as cause and consequence, for much of the available research is not designed to ascertain with confidence what, if anything, caused changes (for example, what causes the state of one's health or how satisfied one is with care). Frequently, a researcher knows that two variables are associated, but is not at all sure that one is responsible for the other. However, in what are called true experiments one gains such confidence, because in these studies the researcher determines who will and who will not receive different experimental treatments (also called interventions). An experiment is designed so that only the special treatment or the intervention could be responsible for subsequent changes in health or behavior.

Numerous experiments have demonstrated that talk can be changed, and that talk can have powerful effects in the medical visit. This research has also shown that it can be surprisingly simple and inexpensive to engineer these changes. This is an extremely important point. If beneficial changes come only with major attitudinal overhauls, extensive training or education, lots of extra attention from research or clinical personnel, or expensive reorganization of the structure of care, then the chances of such interventions ever finding their way into everyday attitudes, medical education, and routine clinical practice are extremely slight.

The interventions discussed below addressed common and everyday problems of patients and physicians, were all relatively straightforward and simple, and yet had impressive results.

INTERVENTION STUDIES WITH PATIENTS

In the actual study from which we extracted the case of the hypothetical gentleman awaiting surgery, some coronary bypass patients' roommates had not yet undergone surgery (as in the example), whereas others had already had their operations (Kulik & Mahler, 1987). If the roommate was *postoperative*, the patient awaiting surgery was significantly less anxious prior to surgery, according to a combined measure of self-rated anxiety, nurse-rated anxiety, and number of tranquilizing medications taken in the two days before surgery. Remarkably, the beneficial effects did not end there. These patients walked more in the first three days after surgery and left the hospital a full

1.4 days sooner than patients whose roommates before surgery were also preoperative.

How could such a simple thing make such a difference? The answer is that under conditions of uncertainty, people look around for clues as to how to react and feel, emotionally and physically. In this study, patients must have looked to their roommates for clues as to how anxious to feel. Because the postoperative roommates were undoubtedly less anxious than they had been before the operation, the patients awaiting surgery were less anxious too. These patients probably gained relief from knowledge that the roommates had survived and seemed generally in one piece. The patients may also have learned from their postoperative roommates particular kinds of information that helped them prepare for the experience—what exactly happened, what it felt like, and so forth (Kulik & Mahler, 1987).

Indeed, a wealth of research demonstrates the beneficial effects of pre-paredness on coping and recovery. This preparedness comes from both factual knowledge about one's medical condition and about what to expect, and from reassurance and support provided by care providers or others at crucial points in a medical crisis. One mechanism whereby information produces positive health effects is the enhanced sense of control that comes when one is able to predict what will happen. Feeling in control of events and circumstances has wide-ranging effects in both the health domain and in other aspects of everyday life. People who feel they have control can better tolerate pain and bodily symptoms. They report fewer health problems, have better health status, and recover more quickly from illness.

In a review of thirty-four controlled experiments that tested the effects of psychological interventions (mostly information and preparation for proce-dures) on patients recovering from surgery or heart attack, it was found that 85% of the effects were beneficial, including an average reduction in hospi-talization of two days. The remaining studies found that interventions made no difference, but caused no harm (Mumford, Schlesinger, & Glass, 1982).

The authors note that the interventions they reviewed covered a range of activities performed by psychiatrists, psychologists, surgeons, anesthesiolo-gists, nurses, and others. The activities were sometimes elaborate special programs, but often were quite simple and inexpensive modifications of standard medical procedures. A typical study included in the review de-scribed the experience of a group of male preoperative patients given the opportunity to meet in a small group led by a nurse the evening before surgery. The participants discussed concerns and fears about the surgery and also heard about what to expect and how to aid in their own recuperation. Compared to comparable control group patients who underwent similar surgery, the experimental group patients slept better, were less anxious the morning of surgery, required less anesthesia and pain medication, suffered less postoperative urinary retention, returned more rapidly to oral intake, and were discharged sooner from the hospital (Schmitt & Woolridge, 1973).

In some studies, the preparedness intervention was not even with the patient—children undergoing tonsillectomy and adenoidectomy—but was with the patient's parent (Mahaffy, 1965). In this case, the intervention had dramatic effects even when filtered through the patients' mothers. The mothers received two brief sessions with a nurse designed to provide information and support. The first session was upon admission to the hospital and the second when the child returned from the recovery room. Children of mothers receiving the intervention were better able to drink liquids, had less vomiting, and cried less during the hospital stay. A follow-up questionnaire completed at home by the child's mother also found much better outcomes for the intervention group. Children of prepared mothers were reported to have had less fever, less disturbed sleep, and less fear of doctors and nurses. The mothers also reported fewer doctor visits to the home during the recovery period.

We can speculate that a mother who is informed and whose anxieties are relieved will explain things better and will behave in a more relaxed and optimistic way, conveying to her child that things are going fine, that it's not so scary, and that she's not worried.

The positive effects of providing information to patients as a means of reducing stress outside the hospital setting have also been demonstrated (Fuller, Endress, & Johnson, 1978; Johnson & Leventhal, 1974; Johnson, Kirchoff, & Endress, 1975). The bulk of these studies assessed the effect of information and preparedness as a means of reducing stress related to unpleasant medical examinations, such as endoscopy, removal of orthopedic casts, or pelvic exams, and demonstrated the wide potential use of information techniques in office settings.

Now we can tell more about the woman we introduced earlier, who lives in a nursing home. The nursing home administrator told her and her floormates not only that they should decide on the appearance of their rooms, but that they should decide on many details of their daily lives—when and whom to visit on the floor, when to watch television, which movies they would like. He invited them to suggest changes to the staff, and then offered them each a houseplant that would be their responsibility.

In this well-known research, the nursing home patients were followed for over a year, as were those on a different floor who were addressed by their administrator but not reminded of the various choices they could make or of the need to take responsibility for themselves (Langer & Rodin, 1976; Rodin & Langer, 1977). Rather, he emphasized that it was the nursing home's responsibility to keep them happy and well cared for. He covered all the same topics, and he gave them a plant, but he did not focus on choice and responsibility.

The results of this study were as dramatic as the intervention was subtle. Patients in the responsibility-induced group became happier, more active, more alert, and improved in health; they spent more time talking with staff and fellow patients; and they had a death rate of 15% in the eighteen months following the intervention, compared to a death rate of 30% in the comparison group.

There can be no doubt that a large share of these effects stemmed from processes internal to the patient. People's capacities are largely determined by what they expect those capacities to be. The will to live is now a confirmed notion in medicine.

In addition, the patients who now talked more to staff and to other patients were probably pleased with the positive effect their interactions had on others' attitudes toward them, which further enhanced self-esteem and the sense of meaningful belonging to a group. And talking more to medical or nursing staff surely had specific effects on the process of medical care: we would bet that experimental patients got better medical care, although this was not assessed in the study. They may have gotten more information, more reassurance, and more attention to their complaints.

Other research has probed more deeply into exactly how doctor-patient communication is affected when patients take a more active role. Earlier, in Chapter 6, we briefly described a study designed to help patients ask questions before entering the doctor's office (Roter, 1977). This was a simple intervention that took about ten minutes in the waiting room prior to the patient's visit with the doctor. The session was structured so that a health educator, together with the patient, would work through a question-asking protocol to identify questions the patient may have about his or her illness or treatment. The protocol was structured to review possible questions in the areas of disease etiology, symptom duration, severity of illness, prevention and lifestyle-related suggestions, and treatment, including medications, diet, and physical therapy (Table 6.1 in Chapter 6 outlines this protocol).

An example of a typical exchange between the health educator and the patient going through the protocol would be:

Educator: Sometimes people forget to take their medicine. Do you have any questions about what you should do if you missed taking your medicine?

Patient: I sometimes wonder about that. I'm not sure whether I should double the dose the next time or just skip it altogether.

Educator: Would you like to ask your doctor about that?

Patient: Yes, I would.

Educator: Tell me exactly how you would ask the doctor your question and I'll
write it down on this piece of paper for you to take into your visit so you won't
forget it when you see your doctor.

Patient: What do I do if I forget to take my medicine—is it OK to just skip it or do
I really need to double the dose the next time? Actually what I really want to
know is what harm there is if I don't take my medicine every single time. You
see, I really think I take too much and, well, I like to give myself a little break
once in awhile, you know, to give my body a rest.

Educator: It sounds like you have several good questions about your medication.
Let's list each question separately.

Patient: OK, first: If I miss a dose of medicine do I just forget it or do I double up
on the next dose? Also, isn't it a good idea to give your body a rest from
medicine every once in awhile?

Educator: (Writes down the questions and reads it back to the patient.) Are these
your questions?

Patient: Yes, these are things I really want to know about.

Educator: Is there anything else you would like to ask your doctor concerning
medicines?

Patient: No, that's it.

If the patient indicated that he or she had no questions in a particular area,
the educator would proceed to the next area. After covering the entire
protocol the educator would read back the list of questions and close the
session by assuring the patient that the questions identified were important,
and encouraging the patient to ask the questions of the doctor.

This process did not produce long lists of questions: patients receiving the
intervention identified slightly less than two questions, on average. However,
this was enough to produce changes in the way patients viewed themselves
and in the communication process. As part of the study, patients' locus of
control was measured. This is a measure that reflects the tendency for
individuals to see themselves as either powerless and at the mercy of destiny,
luck, or other people, or powerful and responsible for their own good or bad
fortune. Someone's sense of control is subject to change based on their
experience, and we found that patients who participated in the intervention
underwent such a change in attitude and self-image. They felt more in control
and responsible for their health, and they acted on these feelings by being
more active in the medical visit and asking more questions. Analysis of tape
recordings of the visits found that the number of questions patients asked
during the medical visit doubled for those participating in the intervention,
compared to a control group. Moreover, during the next six months, intervention group patients more consistently kept appointments with their doctors to monitor their health than those in the control group.

Greenfield and colleagues went even farther in trying to activate patients (Greenfield, Kaplan, & Ware, 1985). These researchers experimented with a group of patients with peptic ulcer disease who attended a Veteran's Administration hospital clinic. During the twenty minutes immediately preceding the medical visit, half the patients were approached by a clinic assistant, who did the following things:

- reviewed the patient's medical record with the patient
- acquainted the patient with how his or her disease is treated at that clinic
- taught the patient a few skills designed to increase the patient's involvement in the doctor-patient interaction

These skills were not elaborate. As the authors write:

Patients were encouraged to ask questions, recognize relevant medical decisions, and negotiate these decisions with physicians. Assistants also coached patients in the use of simple techniques for overcoming common barriers to discussing issues with physicians including embarrassment, fear of appearing foolish, forgetting to bring up an issue, and intimidation by the physician. (Greenfield, Kaplan, & Ware, 1985, p. 521)

The investigators then tape-recorded the visit and gathered postvisit questionnaires from patients and doctors, including a mailed questionnaire nearly two months later. The audiotapes showed that the activated patients, those who got the twenty-minute session (instead of twenty minutes of education just on ulcer disease, which the other half of the patients got), were 30% more active in the conversation with the doctor, were much more assertive, and elicited twice the number of factual statements from the doctor.

Activated patients also reported significantly fewer physical limitations in the weeks that followed the visit, and less limitation on their ability to work and perform other important social roles. The more active they were in the visit (talking more, asking more questions, being more assertive), the better was their reported health later. And the patients seemed to like this new role, for they expressed a significantly stronger preference for active involvement in medical decision making.

This same research team replicated these study findings in a number of additional patient populations, including patients with hypertension, diabetes, and cancer (Kaplan, Greenfield, & Ware, 1989). In separate clinical trials conducted with patients of different socioeconomic and ethnic backgrounds, the researchers found convincingly similar results. As reported with the ulcer patients, hypertensive patients receiving the activation intervention had improved quality of life and functional status ratings, as well as lowered blood pressure during the follow-up period. Diabetic patients demonstrated all the positive effects described earlier, as well as lowered blood glucose upon follow-up, indicating better control of their diabetic condition. The experience of breast cancer patients also paralleled the others. In this case, symptom experience was monitored through patients' diaries and found to lessen for intervention group patients over the course of chemotherapy.

What is intriguingly similar about the Greenfield et al. studies and those of Langer and Rodin, besides their dramatic results, is that patients receiving the intervention talked more with their providers. In the Greenfield studies the talk was explicitly related to the patient's medical agenda for improved health, while in the other the talk was more general in nature. Although neither study looked closely at how care providers reacted, either in terms of dialogue or in terms of the technical quality of care, it is certainly possible that the benefits of the intervention came from both. We expect that improved care came from better quality of care, as well as from the patient feeling more in control.

For some patients a greater feeling of control may come with confidence that they are fully informed of all important information without fear of being left in the dark, either purposely or by accident. This issue is perhaps most pressing for patients with very serious illnesses like cancer. For instance, a study of cancer patients by Fallowfield and associates (Fallowfield, Baum, & Maguire, 1986) found that more than half the patients felt that the information the doctor gave to them at the "bad news" visit had been inadequate. Most of these patients acknowledged, however, that the diagnosis of cancer had so shocked or stunned them that they were unable to recall very much of the rest of the conversation.

Fallowfield and her colleagues started a unique program to deal with this problem. All patients during the study period coming to a general surgical outpatient department for a consultation concerning their diagnosis and treatment were asked for permission to audiotape the medical visit. Forty-six patients with a diagnosis of either bowel or breast cancer participated in the study. At the end of the medical visit, the patients were invited to take the recording of the visit home with them, along with a questionnaire that assessed the tape's usefulness (Hogbin & Fallowfield, 1989).

Virtually all of the patients reported listening to the tape, and said that it was useful on several levels. Patients indicated that the audiotape was helpful in clarifying points of confusion and reminding them of forgotten information, that it served to reassure and calm them, and that the audiotape made it easier for them to convey the distressing information to family and friends. Some of the comments, as reported by patients on the questionnaires, are especially telling. One patient noted: "I found the tape very helpful indeed for the reasons below: (1) it prevented me from unintentionally distorting any information I was given; (2) the calm and factual discussion is very useful to listen to again at times of panic and despair." Another patient noted to the doctor, "Your idea of the tape was brilliant, as I found I couldn't tell my family. They found it very helpful and put their minds at rest. Your tape gave me great comfort and confidence in you."

Although the original study did not follow up patients to measure long-term consequences, it is easy to foresee changes in future interactions between these patients and their doctors. A patient who has truly heard distressing and often very complicated information about his or her medical condition, as opposed to patients who feel they are in the dark, is likely to feel more knowledgeable, ask more intelligent questions, be treated more as a partner, and will likely adopt a more directive role in his or her own medical care in subsequent medical visits. As we know, these effects are not just beneficial in themselves; they are related to improvements in coping, health, and mortality.

These same researchers are currently conducting a clinical trial to determine psychological and coping effects associated with provision of an audiotape of the "bad news" visit, and anticipate changes along all of the dimensions just mentioned.

Another way to give patients assurance that they have all the information they need is to give them the medical record (Bronson, Costanza, & Tufo, 1986). This would have been helpful to the elderly gentleman, mentioned in our third vignette, who was unsure of important facts regarding his health and medical regimen. In this study, investigators simply mailed elderly patients copies of their physicians' progress notes from the most recent visit (typewritten for legibility). They discovered that patients gained greater understanding of their health problems and their treatments, compared to a group of similar patients in a control group. The investigators didn't follow up the patients at the next medical visit, but again, we believe there would be significant differences in the way these patients participate in their care.

PHYSICIAN INTERVENTIONS

It can be argued that physicians are a much more efficient target of interventions designed to change doctor-patient communication than are patients. After all, an intervention that changes a physician's behavior in the medical visit is likely to affect thousands of patients each year. Fortunately, as we have seen with patient interventions, there are fairly simple strategies that can make substantial changes.

Inui and associates developed a single-session training program for doctors designed to improve the compliance of patients with high blood pressure (Inui, Yourtee, & Williamson, 1976). The training included a one-time teaching session (one to two hours in length) given to a randomly selected group of internal medicine residents. During the session, findings from an earlier study with this same patient population were presented, which documented widespread patient noncompliance with hypertension medications. Simple means of identifying the noncompliant patient were emphasized. For instance, the prior study found that 90% of patients with diastolic pressure greater than 100 mm Hg were likely to be noncompliant. If the patient gave a history of past hospitalization for blood pressure, and had a diastolic pressure greater than 100 mm Hg, the probability of noncompliance was 96%.

The session emphasized the need for physicians to include an analysis of the patient's knowledge, attitudes, and beliefs regarding his or her medical problems as part of the patient's history and physical exam. In fact, the study's approach required that the physicians learn a different doctoring role—one that deemphasized the physician's job as a diagnostician and reemphasized his or her role as a patient educator. Strategies for enhancing patient compliance were reviewed, including the relation of patients' ideas to their perception of the seriousness of hypertension, susceptibility to its complications, and the efficacy of therapy.

The results of the study were dramatic. Trained physicians allocated a greater percentage of visit time to patient education than did control physicians. This resulted in increased patient knowledge and more appropriate patient beliefs regarding hypertension and its therapy. Patients of the trained physicians were more compliant with drug regimens and had better control of blood pressure than control group patients. These changes were still evident six months after the tutorials.

Following Inui's study with internists, Maiman and associates designed a tutorial for pediatricians to enhance patient (mother/child) compliance with antibiotic regimens (Maiman, Becker, Liptak, Nazarian, & Rounds, 1988). All full-time pediatricians in the Rochester, New York, area were invited to participate in the study. Ninety-one agreed, and were randomly assigned to one of three groups; two of these were treatment groups and the third a control group.

The first group received a two-session tutorial totaling five hours, as well as supplemental reading material on pediatric compliance with drug regimens. The tutorial sessions addressed the magnitude and determinants of noncompliance and provided practical compliance-enhancing strategies relevant to regimens for acute and chronic pediatric conditions, both in general terms and specifically in relation to children with otitis media.

Six approaches and techniques for increasing compliance were addressed:

1.   Use of individualized, written instructions to reinforce oral explanations of details of the regimen

2. Reduction of regimen complexity when possible by simplifying dosage and scheduling of drugs

3. Special approaches for regimens requiring changes in lifestyle behaviors

4. Assessment and modification of parent/child health beliefs by addressing relevant perceptions and attitudes

5. Acknowledging the association between satisfaction with pediatrician-mother interaction on compliance and the need to meet the mother's expectations for the visit

6. Stressing the magnitude of noncompliance and ways to monitor the problem

To compare the usefulness of the tutorial with a less expensive alternative, the second group of physicians did not attend the tutorial but received, through the mail, the same reading materials on patient compliance made available to the first group.

Over a six-month period following the intervention, mothers of children with otitis media (ear infection) who were given a ten-day antibiotic regimen were randomly selected by the research staff from the participating pediatricians' appointment rosters. Within eight days of the medical visit a home interview was conducted, in which the mothers were questioned about their doctor's communication behavior during the medical visit. Mothers were also asked about the extent to which they adhered to the full ten-day drug regimen.

Both groups of intervention doctors performed much better than physicians in the control group, but surprisingly, there were few consistent differences between physicians in the two intervention groups. Doctors attending the tutorials used more of the compliance-enhancing strategies than physicians receiving the printed materials, but the differences were not very great. Mothers of children seeing these pediatricians were found to be much better compliers with the prescribed antibiotic regimens than patients of control group physicians. Furthermore, these effects appeared to be long-lasting. Patients who enrolled late in the study, that is up to six months after the physicians received the tutorials or reading material, showed the same positive effects as patients followed early in the study period.

The investigators conclude that the much simpler intervention, sending relevant material in the mail to doctors, with its lower cost and greater practicability, deserves consideration as part of a continuing medical education curriculum for practicing pediatricians.

As successful as the interventions described above were, they suffered from the limitation of attempting to change the interaction between two people by intervening with only one person. We wonder how much more effective these experiments might have been had both patients and their doctors received the same kinds of intervention, reinforcing and emphasizing the same message.

One study that prepared both doctors and patients for the visit was undertaken by Jacobs and associates (Jacobs, Carols, Jacobs, Weinstein, & Mann, 1972). The preparation was subtle, and neither the doctors nor the patients realized that they were part of a study. For the physicians (psychiatrists), the experimental intervention consisted of a few extra minutes embedded in the usual briefing a doctor received regarding a psychiatric walk-in patient, and included a short talk on the needs and expectations of poor and uneducated patients in undergoing psychiatric treatment. For patients, the preparation was simply being told that talking with a psychiatrist is different from talking with other doctors—a psychiatrist will try to get to the root of trouble by talking over emotional problems.

Preparation for the visit was a marked success: it increased the doctor's display of interest in the patient, the development of a treatment plan, and the doctor's seeing the patient on an ongoing basis. Furthermore, prepared patients were rated by the doctors as more improved. When patients and doctors did not receive preparation, the patients were viewed more pessimistically by the doctors than patients in the other groups, they had worse prognoses, were more heavily medicated, and dropped out of care more frequently.

How is it that these doctors needed to be reminded to talk to their patients? A study of the process by which interns and residents learn how to cure patients, but forget how to care for them, makes a frightening indictment of the educational process (Mizrahi, 1986). As discussed in Chapter 4, terrible pressure is put on these young doctors, and getting rid of patients—spending the least amount of time possible and discharging the patient at the earliest moment—becomes the paramount goal. In the process, negative stereotypes of patients are compounded and reinforced. Reading about the world Mizrahi observed fills one with great pessimism: our best and brightest young doctors are being trained out of the idealism and natural talent that drew them to medicine in the first place.

An often-quoted study by Helfer (1970) brings this point home. Helfer found that freshmen medical students obtained significantly more relevant interpersonal information and asked fewer leading questions than senior medical students. The younger students were better at just plain talk. As students moved through their training, a certain degree of their innate ability to communicate seemed to be supplanted by their desire to obtain factual information in an attempt to test biomedical hypotheses. This alteration limited their effectiveness as good doctors. For the most part, these students learned interviewing skills by imitating their clinical teachers, who were also more likely to value the collection of facts over less constrained communication.

This unfortunate course of events is not inevitable, however. For example, a study of Israeli medical students and their physician mentors speaks to this point. These students participated in ten ninety-minute sessions on interviewing skills, held twice a week for five weeks (Kramer, Ber, & Moore, 1987). At these meetings the students talked about admitting a patient to the hospital, diagnosing a life-threatening disease, death and dying, teamwork, uncertainty, and chronic disease. In addition, time was taken for role playing, with the students and mentors playing the roles of patients, physicians, and family members. The students' and physicians' "rejecting behavior" was studied both before and after in visits with real patients. Rejecting behavior included sarcasm, contempt, verbal rejection, nonresponsiveness to the patient's statements, and evading eye contact.

The results showed that before training the medical students engaged in much less rejection than did the physicians. Students averaged about six negative behaviors per interview before training, while physicians averaged almost twice as many. One year after training, students engaged in an average of two rejective behaviors, and physicians in five. A control group of students who did not receive training averaged eleven rejecting behaviors. Thus, negativity was substantially lower for both medical students and physicians, even after a year, while members of the control group increased rejecting behaviors over time.

This study underscores the damage that physicians can do as role models to their students, and what the natural toll of increasing responsibility may be on medical students over time. Medical students imitate their clinical teachers' patterns of dealing with patients. If the teachers exhibit a dehumanized and rejecting pattern of communication with patients, the students learn that pattern. On a positive note, it is clear that the damage done to the young medical student's ability and inclination to be compassionate and empathetic can be prevented, diminished, or undone. Further, it is reassuring to see that even well-respected and established physicians can change longstanding patterns of communication for the better.

Just as treating patients in a rejecting manner is hurtful to the patient, so is the lack of empathetic behaviors. But again, studies show that empathy can be improved in both medical students and experienced doctors (Kalisch, 1971; Fine & Therrien, 1977). For instance, doctors trained in empathy can improve their ability to indicate understanding and offer feelings, make eye contact, appear more attentive and interested, and encourage their patients to talk more.

The findings from these studies are encouraging, in that many critics of interviewing skills training maintain that while medical students' behavior may be amenable to change, physicians already practicing in the community have an entrenched interviewing style. This is not the case, as reflected in the Israeli study just mentioned, or in our own work. We designed a study to develop and evaluate a continuing medical education program for community-based, primary care physicians with the hope to improve their recognition and address of patients' psychosocial problems. Sixty-nine doctors and 652 of their patients participated in the study. The study physicians were randomly assigned to one of two eight-hour interviewing skills groups (emphasizing handling emotions or problem solving), or to a nontreatment control group. The skills groups met twice, one week apart, for two four-hour sessions. Most of the time was spent in small groups of three to five physicians, with a preceptor experienced in teaching interviewing skills and a simulated patient to assist in role playing. Table 9.1 displays key elements of the training curriculum.

The success of our teaching program was evaluated by going to the offices of all study physicians and tape recording them with a number of their actual patients. (Of course, both patients and physicians were aware of the study and consented to tape recording of the visits.) Since we were particularly interested in how the doctors dealt with emotionally distressed patients, we administered a standardized measure of patient distress, the General Health Questionnaire (GHQ), to all study patients. In this way we were able to tell which patients were likely to be suffering from mental distress and which were not, and analyze the audiotapes of an equal number of each type patient.

All of the patients found to be distressed according to the screening questionnaire were called by telephone at two weeks, three months, and six months after the medical visit to assess health status—both physical and mental.

We found that the trained physicians did indeed use significantly more of the trained behaviors during the medical visits than control group physicians, and there were relatively few differences in performance between the two trained groups. We also found significant differences by treatment group in physicians' ability to identify patients in emotional distress. Trained physicians were better than control group physicians at recognizing which of their patients were distressed.

Long-term effects of the intervention were also evident. Patients of trained doctors showed significantly greater improvement in their mental health than the control group patients up to six months following the medical visit.

We agree with Mumford and colleagues:

In an action-oriented society, reports of the considerable effectiveness of modest interventions may command less attention than reports of the modest effects of more

Table 9.1
Critical Communication Skills for the Physician

I. Elicit the Full Spectrum of Patient Concerns

    A. *Use open-ended questions*
    Example: What's been going on since I saw you last?

    B. *Resist immediate follow-up*
    Example: I know you came in to have your mole checked. Is there anything else that is bothering you or causing you concern that you would like to discuss today?

    C. *Set priorities by negotiating an agenda and use of time*
    Examples:

      • Of all these problems, which do you consider the most troubling?

      • There are a number of important things for us to work on. Which of these would you like to tackle today, and which could be taken up at our next visit?

II. Explore the Significance and Impact of the Problem

    A. *Ask explicitly for the patient's opinion, experience, understanding, and interpretation*
    Examples:

      • What do you think your problem is?

      • Has anything like this happened before?

      • What do you think caused it?

      • What do you think it means?

      • What troubles you most about it?

    B. *Ask explicitly for expectations*
    Example: What do you think I can do that would help?

III. Effectively Eliciting and Responding to Patient Emotions

    A. *Ask for feelings*
    Examples:

      • How do you feel about that?

      • What are your concerns?

      • Are you worried about anything related to this (condition)?

B. *Compliment patient effort*
Example: I want you to know that I think you are doing a good job managing this complicated regimen.

C. *Legitimate the patient's feelings*
Example: I would be surprised if a person with your problem did not feel angry.

D. *Express accurate empathy*
Verbal examples:

- You seem really anxious about this.

- You look worried (angry, anxious, hesitant, etc.).

Nonverbal examples: Forward lean of the body; using a sad or sympathetic tone of voice; showing a concerned or distressed facial expression. Physical contact (such as putting an arm around a patient's shoulder, squeezing a hand, or patting an arm) can enhance empathy, but should be used with care as patients show wide variation in their responses to uninvited physical contact.

flamboyant interventions. It is often argued that the medical care system cannot afford to take on the emotional status of the patient as its responsibility. Time is short and costs are high. However, it may be that medicine cannot afford to ignore the patient's emotional status assuming that it will take care of itself. (Mumford, Schlesinger, & Glass, 1982, p. 144)

We would like to close this chapter with a description of doctors and patients connecting in a fundamental and meaningful way, written by Anthony Suchman and Dale Matthews (1988).

These physicians are among a growing group who have participated in interviewing skills training that includes not only practice of the kinds of skills represented in the studies above, but also an emphasis on self-awareness and personal growth as part of the educational process. This curriculum is being developed as part of a national effort to improve the medical interview (Lipkin, Quill, & Napodano, 1984). Workshops are held annually that bring together recognized leaders in primary care internal medicine to teach their skills to other physicians who, in turn, teach medical students.

Suchman and Matthews write:

A family doctor returns to his office to find a desk covered with messages: "Joyce wants you to call as soon as you are back"; "Call Joyce's husband ASAP—wants to know why she needs blood"; and, "Joyce called again—don't forget to see her." The patient is a 38-year-old woman, who is a mid-level executive in a local firm, and a mother of two. Two weeks after a protracted evaluation, she was diagnosed as having Hodgkin's disease, a very serious and often fatal form of cancer. "Why do I need a transfusion?" she demands as the doctor enters her hospital room. "With my luck, I'll get hepatitis." The doctor tells her that the surgical team ordered that her blood type be identified, but not that she receive a transfusion. "Well, a person came around to draw more blood this afternoon. I asked why they need more when they already took several tubes this morning. She told me that it was for a blood transfusion, and I started to get the feeling that nobody was telling me what's going on around here." With pursed lips and arms folded tightly across her chest, the patient looked like she was ready for a fight.

The doctor put together the phone messages, the worry about hepatitis, the frustration and anxiety of her protracted diagnostic evaluation and present body language, and realized how much more frightened she was than she wished to show, or know. "This has been a hard day for you, hasn't it?" The patient's shoulders sagged and she lowered her head for a moment and then looked up at the doctor, her eyes filling with tears. The doctor could feel her fears of a painful postoperative recovery, of her children without a mother, and losing her ability to work. But even more, the doctor sensed dismay. Joyce had been trying so hard to remain in control and to hide fears from herself and from her husband who was on the threshold of panic. She realized how desperate and exaggerated her response to the unexpected blood work had been, she recognized the underlying panic of her own that this belied.

In that next moment, patient and doctor completely shared those feelings of worry and dismay, and it was immensely meaningful to both. It was a moment of special closeness and intimacy; it was an expression of the very healing bond that makes medicine art and magic. "There are no heroes here," the doctor said, taking her hand, "just people." (Suchman & Matthews, 1988, p. 125)

REFERENCES

Bronson, D. L., Costanza, M. C., & Tufo, H. M. (1986). Using medical records for older patient education in ambulatory practice. *Medical Care, 24*, 332–339.

Fallowfield, L. J., Baum, M., & Maguire, G. P. (1986). Effects of breast conservation on psychological morbidity associated with diagnosis and treatment of early breast cancer. *British Medical Journal, 293*, 1331–1334.

Fine, V. K., & Therrien, M. E. (1977). Empathy in the doctor-patient relationship: Skill training for medical students. *Journal of Medical Education, 52*, 152–157.

Fuller, S., Endress, P. L., & Johnson, J. (1978, December). The effects of cognitive and behavioral control on coping with an aversive health examination. *Journal of Human Stress*, 18–25.

Greenfield, S., Kaplan, S., & Ware, J. E., Jr. (1985). Expanding patient involvement in care: Effects on patient outcomes. *Annals of Internal Medicine, 102*, 520–528.

Helfer, R. E. (1970). An objective comparison of the pediatric interviewing skills of freshman and senior medical students. *Pediatrics, 45*, 623–627.

Hogbin, B., & Fallowfield, L. (1989). Getting it taped: The "bad news" consultation with cancer patients. *British Journal of Hospital Medicine, 41*, 330–333.

Inui, T. S., Yourtee, E. L., & Williamson, J. W. (1976). Improved outcomes in hypertension after physician tutorials: A controlled trial. *Annals of Internal Medicine, 84,* 646–651.

Jacobs, D., Carols, E., Jacobs, T., Weinstein, H., & Mann, D. (1972). Preparation for treatment of the disadvantaged patient: Effects on disposition and outcome. *American Journal of Orthopsychiatry, 42,* 666–673.

Johnson, J., Kirchoff, K., & Endress, P. (1975). Altering childrens' distress behavior during orthopedic cast removal. *Nursing Research, 24,* 404–410.

Johnson, J., & Leventhal, H. (1974). Effects of accurate expectations and behavioral instructions on reactions during a noxious medical examination. *Journal of Personality and Social Psychology, 29,* 710–718.

Kalisch, B. J. (1971). An experiment in the development of empathy in nursing students. *Nursing Research, 20,* 202–210.

Kaplan, S. H., Greenfield, S., & Ware, J. E., Jr. (1989). Assessing the effects of physician-patient interactions on the outcomes of chronic disease. *Medical Care, 27,* S110–S127.

Kramer, D., Ber, R., & Moore, M. (1987). Impact of workshop on students' and physicians' rejecting behaviors in patient interview. *Journal of Medical Education, 62,* 904–910.

Kulik, J. A., & Mahler, H.T.M. (1987). Effects of preoperative roommate assignment on preoperative anxiety and recovery from coronary-bypass surgery. *Health Psychology, 6,* 525–543.

Langer, E. J., & Rodin, J. (1976). The effects of choice and enhanced personal responsibility for the aged: A field experiment in an institutional setting. *Journal of Personality and Social Psychology, 34,* 191–198.

Lipkin, M., Jr., Quill, T. E., & Napodano, R. J. (1984). The medical interview: A curriculum for residencies in internal medicine. *Annals of Internal Medicine, 100,* 277–284.

Mahaffy, P. R. (1965). The effects of hospitalization on children admitted for tonsillectomy and adenoidectomy. *Nursing Research, 14,* 12–19.

Maiman, L. A., Becker, M. H., Liptak, G. S., Nazarian, L. F., & Rounds, K. A. (1988). Improving pediatricians' compliance-enhancing practices: A randomized trial. *American Journal of Diseases of Children, 142,* 773–779.

Mizrahi, T. (1986). *Getting rid of patients: Contradictions in the socialization of physicians.* New Brunswick, N.J.: Rutgers University Press.

Mumford, E., Schlesinger, H. J., & Glass, G.V. (1982). The effects of psychological intervention on recovery from surgery and heart attacks: An analysis of the literature. *American Journal of Public Health, 72,* 141–151.

Rodin, J., & Langer, E. J. (1977). Long-term effects of a control-relevant intervention with the institutionalized aged. *Journal of Personality and Social Psychology, 35,* 897–902.

Roter, D. (1977). Patient participation in the patient-provider interaction: The effects of patient question asking on the quality of interaction, satisfaction, and compliance. *Health Education Monographs, 5,* 281–315.

Schmitt, F. E., & Woolridge, P. J. (1973). Psychological preparation of surgical patients. *Nursing Research, 22,* 108–116.

Suchman, A. L., & Matthews, D. A. (1988). What makes the patient-doctor relationship therapeutic?: Exploring the connexional dimension of medical care. *Annals of Internal Medicine, 108,* 125–130.

Part IV
Conclusions

10

Toward a Healthier Medical Visit

Discussion between doctors and patients has long been regarded as the way in which much of the curing and caring of medicine is conveyed. Sometimes regarded as the art or heart of medicine, its importance is well noted in antiquity and recognized in modern times. However, only since the mid-1960s have the actual dynamics of the therapeutic dialogue been observed in any systematic manner, bringing the opportunity to recast this aspect of medicine as science rather than as art, intuition, or anecdote. These studies tell us about what happens between doctors and patients, and about the significance of these events for attitudes, feelings, and for health itself. The interpersonal aspects of medical care are now known to be as much, or sometimes even more, an "active ingredient" as are the pills and other treatments given to patients.

If we were challenged to summarize the key messages of our book we would outline three. First, we believe that the therapeutic potential of medicine can be enhanced—diagnosis made more accurate, treatment more effective, recovery faster and less painful, and quality of life more fully realized. And, the vehicle by which this will be accomplished is the doctor-patient relationship.

Second, we believe that both doctors and patients can change the nature of their relationship and its interaction through modest interventions with far-reaching consequences. This is not to say that the determinants of behavior are simple. We have reviewed a great deal of research attesting to the complex effects of previous experience and culture on behavior; however, we are confident in our conclusion that the doctor-patient relationship is remarkably sensitive to efforts at change.

Finally, we believe that responsibility for change lies with both patients and physicians. However, each actor alone in the relationship has the power to transform the way in which the script of the medical visit is written. We have seen in our review of work that interventions directed toward patients, but without provider involvement, have been effective in achieving significant changes in the way in which the visit is conducted. Likewise, programs designed to change physician behavior have led to dramatic differences in the communication of the visit. We believe interventions would be all the more successful if they were to address simultaneously both of the participants in the medical encounter.

The most successful patient interventions foster and encourage a partnership between patients and physicians—a partnership based on patients' confidence in their own self-knowledge and ability to take an active and competent role in their own medical affairs. For physicians we believe that the most effective interventions are also those that foster a partnership based on an acknowledgment of the unique store of experience and insight possessed by the patient, which can be as crucial for a positive treatment outcome as the physician's biomedical knowledge. There is a need for physicians to recognize that "apples are red and sweet as well as being composed of cells and molecules" (White, 1988, p. 6)—that the patient's experience of life is more than the function of body systems.

The medical community is of two minds when considering issues of the doctor-patient relationship. The centrality of the doctor-patient relationship to patient care is among the oldest of themes in the history of medicine, dating back to the time of Hippocrates. Public concern for the quality of the therapeutic relationship is no less great in modern times. Indeed, this concern has led to at least token acknowledgment in that some course dealing with this topic has been incorporated into the curriculum of most major medical schools. Yet for many physicians technology and the scientific method, divorced from issues of the therapeutic relationship, are viewed as the sine qua non of medicine. In the real practice of medicine, many maintain, the issue of the doctor-patient relationship is an inconsequential and unscientific, low-priority concern.

Nonetheless, we end this book with optimism. There are many indications that the doctor-patient relationship is undergoing evolution. It is a "moving target" with a dynamic nature. As reflected in the landmark work *The Task of Medicine: Dialogue at Wickenburg* (White, 1988), a growing cadre of influential physicians in mainstream American medicine have taken the lead in studying communication processes and teaching other physicians about them; as mentors and role models, such physician-teachers will change the attitudes and knowledge of the next generation. Medical educators as well as medical researchers now freely acknowledge the limits of their own training and experience, and invite nonphysicians—health educators, psychologists, sociologists—to join in the training of doctors and in research on the processes of effective medical care. The psychology of health and illness is now a well-studied topic in schools of public health and medicine and in departments of psychology in many American universities. Change is imminent.

Some people yearn for the good old days when doctors really knew their patients, made house calls, and had the undying respect of those whom they served. But this idealized past, we believe, will give way to a future doctor-patient relationship in which true respect will characterize the exchange, collaboration will replace medical authority, and the wisdom of both biomedical and social science will be applied to preserving that delicate balance we call health.

REFERENCE

White, K. L. (1988). *The task of medicine: Dialogue at Wickenburg.* Menlo Park, Calif.: Henry J. Kaiser Family Foundation.

Bibliography

American Medical Association, Special Task Force on Professional Liability and Insurance. (1984–85). Professional liability in the 1980s.

Aries, E. (1987). Gender and communication. In Shaver, P., & Hendrick, C. (Eds.), *Review of personality and social psychology*, vol.7. Newbury Park, Calif.: Sage Publications.

Asch, D., & Parker, R. (1988). The Libby Zion case. *New England Journal of Medicine, 318*, 771–774.

Bain, D. J. (1976). Doctor-patient communication in general practice consultations. *Medical Education, 10*, 125–131.

Bain, D. J. (1977). Patient knowledge and the content of the consultation in general practice. *Medical Education, 11*, 347–350.

Bain, D. J. (1979). The content of physician/patient communication in family practice. *Journal of Family Practice, 8*, 745–753.

Barber, B. (1980). *Informed consent in medical therapy and research*. New Brunswick, N.J.: Rutgers University Press.

Barzini, L. (1965). *The Italians*. New York: Bantam Press.

Beckman, H. B., & Frankel, R. M. (1984). The effect of physician behavior on the collection of data. *Annals of Internal Medicine, 101*, 692–696.

Beckman, H. B., Frankel, R. M., & Darnley, J. (1985). Soliciting the patient's complete agenda: A relationship to the distribution of concerns. *Clinical Research, 33*, 714A.

Beisecker, A. E., & Beisecker, T. D. (1990). Patient information-seeking behaviors when communicating with doctors. *Medical Care, 28*, 19–28.

Bensing, J. (1991). *Doctor-patient communication and the quality of care: An observation study into affective and instrumental behavior in general practice*. Utrecht, Netherlands: NIVEL.

Bernstein, B., & Kane, R. (1981). Physicians' attitudes toward female patients. *Medical Care, 19*, 600–608.

Bertakis, K. D., Roter, D., & Putnam, S. M. (1991). The relationship of physician medical interview style to patient satisfaction. *Journal of Family Practice, 32*, 175–181.

Biener, L. (1983). Perceptions of patients by emergency room staff: Substance-abusers vs. non-substance-abusers. *Journal of Health and Social Behavior, 24*, 264–275.

Boreham, P., & Gibson, D. (1978). The informative process in private medical consultations: A preliminary investigation. *Social Science & Medicine, 12*, 409–416.

Bosk, C. L. (1979). *Forgive and remember: Managing medical failure.* Chicago: University of Chicago Press.

Boyd, J. R., Covington, T. R., Stanaszek, W. F., & Coussons, R. T. (1974). Drug defaulting: Part I, Determinants of compliance. *American Journal of Hospital Pharmacy, 31*, 362–366.

Brody, D. S. (1980). The patient's role in clinical decision making. *Annals of Internal Medicine, 93*, 718–722.

Brody, D. S., Miller, S. M., Lerman, C. E., Smith, D. G., & Caputo, G.C. (1989). Patient perception of involvement in medical care: Relationship to illness attitudes and outcomes. *Journal of General Internal Medicine, 4*, 506–511.

Bronson, D. L., Costanza, M. C., & Tufo, H. M. (1986). Using medical records for older patient education in ambulatory practice. *Medical Care, 24*, 332–339.

Buller, M. K., & Buller, D. B. (1985). Physicians' communication style and patient satisfaction. *Journal of Health and Social Behavior, 28*, 375–388.

Butterfield, P. (1988). The stress of residency: A review of the literature. *Archives of Internal Medicine, 148*, 1428–1435.

Byrne, P. S., & Long, B.E.L. (1976). *Doctors talking to patients.* London: Her Majesty's Stationery Office.

Caporael, L. R. (1981). The paralanguage of caregiving: Baby talk to the institutionalized aged. *Journal of Personality and Social Psychology, 40*, 876–884.

Caporael, L. R., Lukaszewski, M. P., & Culbertson, G. H. (1983). Secondary baby talk: Judgments by institutionalized elderly and their caregivers. *Journal of Personality and Social Psychology, 44*, 746–756.

Cartwright, A. (1964). *Human relations and hospital care.* London: Routledge & Kegan Paul.

Cartwright, A. (1967). *Patients and their doctors.* London: Routledge & Kegan Paul.

Cartwright, A., & Anderson, R. (1981). *General practice revisited: A second study of patients and their doctors.* London: Tavistock Publications.

Cassell, E. J. (1976). *The healer's art.* Cambridge, Mass.: MIT Press.

Cassileth, B. R., Zupkis, R. V., Sutton-Smith, K., & March, V. (1980). Information and participation preferences among cancer patients. *Annals of Internal Medicine, 92*, 832–836.

Christy, N. P. (1979). English is our second language. *New England Journal of Medicine, 300*, 979–981.

Coe, R. M. (1970). *Sociology of medicine.* New York: McGraw-Hill.

Colford, J. M., & McPhee, S. J. (1989). The ravelled sleeve of care: Managing the stresses of residency training. *Journal of the American Medical Association, 261*, 889–893.

Cousins, N. (1979). *Anatomy of an illness as perceived by the patient.* New York: Norton.

Covington, T. R., Porter, M. E., & See, K. (1979). Improper prescription instructions: A factor in patient compliance. *Patient Counselling and Health Education, 1*, 97–100.

Cypress, B. K. (1980). Characteristics of visits to female and male physicians. Vital and Health Statistics, series 13, no. 49. Hyattsville, Md.: U.S. Department of Health and Human Services.

Davis, F. (1972). Uncertainty in medical prognosis, clinical and functional. In Freidson, E., & Lorber, J. (Eds.), *Medical men and their work: A sociological reader.* Chicago: Aldine Atherton.

Day, S. C., Norcini, J. J., Shea, J. A., & Benson, J. A., Jr. (1989). Gender differences in the clinical competence of residents in internal medicine. *Journal of General Internal Medicine, 4*, 309–312.

DiMatteo, M. R. (1979). Nonverbal skill and the physician-patient relationship. In Rosenthal, R. (Ed.), *Skill in nonverbal communication: Individual differences.* Cambridge, Mass.: Oelgeschlager, Gunn & Hain.

DiMatteo, M. R., & DiNicola, D. D. (1982). *Achieving patient compliance.* New York: Pergamon Press.

DiMatteo, M. R., Hays, R. D., & Prince, L. M. (1986). Relationship of physicians' nonverbal communication skill to patient satisfaction, appointment noncompliance, and physician workload. *Health Psychology, 5*, 581–594.

Domenighetti, G., Luraschi, P., Casabianca, A., Gutzwiller, F., Spinelli, A., Pedrinis, E., & Repetto, F. (1988). Effect of information campaign by the mass media on hysterectomy rates. *The Lancet*, 24–31 December, 1470–1473.

Drew, J., Stoeckle, J. D., & Billings, J. A. (1983). Tips, status and sacrifice: Gift giving in the doctor-patient relationship. *Social Science & Medicine, 17*, 399–404.

Dungal, L. (1978). Physicians' responses to patients: A study of factors involved in the office interview. *Journal of Family Practice, 6*, 1065–1073.

Egbert, L. D., Battit, G. E., Welch, C. E., & Bartlett, M. K. (1964). Reduction of postoperative pain by encouragement and instruction of patients. *New England Journal of Medicine, 270*, 825–827.

Eisenberg, J. M. (1979). Sociologic influences on decision making by clinicians. *Annals of Internal Medicine, 90*, 957–964.

Eisenberg, J. (1986). *Doctors' decisions and the cost of medical care.* Ann Arbor, Mich.: Health Administration Press.

Ende, J., Kazis, L., Ash, A., & Moskowitz, M. A. (1989). Measuring patients'
    desire for autonomy: Decision making and information-seeking prefer-
    ences among medical patients. *Journal of General Internal Medicine, 4*,
    23–30.
Ende, J., Kazis, L., & Moskowitz, M. A. (1990). Preferences for autonomy when
    patients are physicians. *Journal of General Internal Medicine, 5*, 506–509.
Engel, G. L. (1977). The need for a new medical model: A challenge for biomedi-
    cine. *Science, 196*, 129–136.
Epstein, A. M., Begg, C. B., & McNeil, B. J. (1984). The effects of physicians'
    training and personality on test ordering for ambulatory patients. *American
    Journal of Public Health, 74*, 1271–1273.
Epstein, A. M., Begg, C. B., & McNeil, B. J. (1986). The use of ambulatory testing
    in prepaid and fee-for-service group practices: Relation to perceived prof-
    itability. *New England Journal of Medicine, 314*, 1089–1094.
Epstein, A. M., Hall, J. A., Tognetti, J., Son, L. H., & Conant, L., Jr. (1989). Using
    proxies to evaluate quality of life: Can they provide valid information
    about patients' health status and satisfaction with medical care? *Medical
    Care, 27*, S91–S98.
Epstein, A. M., & McNeil, B. J. (1987). Variations in ambulatory test use: What do
    they mean? *Medical Clinics of North America, 71*, 705–717.
Faden, R., Becker, C., Lewis, C., Freeman, J., & Faden, A. (1981). Disclosure of
    information to patients in medical care. *Medical Care, 19*, 718–733.
Fallowfield, L. J., Baum, M., & Maguire, G. P. (1986). Effects of breast conserva-
    tion on psychological morbidity associated with diagnosis and treatment of
    early breast cancer. *British Medical Journal, 293*, 1331–1334.
Fine, V. K., & Therrien, M. E. (1977). Empathy in the doctor-patient relationship:
    Skill training for medical students. *Journal of Medical Education, 52*,
    152–157.
Fischback, R. L., Bayog, A. S., Needle, A., & Delbanco, T. L. (1980). The patient
    and practitioner as co-authors of the medical record. *Patient Counseling
    and Health Education, 2*, 1–5.
Fox, J. G., & Storms, D. M. (1981). A different approach to sociodemographic
    predictors of satisfaction with health care. *Social Science & Medicine, 15A*,
    557–564.
Fox, R. (1989). *Essays in medical sociology: Journeys into the field*. New Bruns-
    wick, N.J.: Transaction Books.
Freeman, S. H. (1987). Health promotion talk in family practice encounters. *Social
    Science & Medicine, 25*, 961-966.
Freidson, E. (1960). Client control and medical practice. *American Journal of
    Sociology, 65*, 374–382.
Freidson, E. (1970a). *Profession of medicine: A study of the sociology of applied
    knowledge*. New York: Dodd Mead.
Freidson, E. (1970b). *Professional dominance*. Chicago: Aldine Press.
Freidson, E. (1975). *Doctoring together: A study of professional social control*.
    New York: Elsevier.

Freire, P. (1970). *Pedagogy of the oppressed*. New York: Seabury Press.

Friedman, H. S., DiMatteo, M. R., & Taranta, A. (1980). A study of the relationship between individual differences in nonverbal expressiveness and factors of personality and social interaction. *Journal of Research in Personality*, *14*, 351–364.

Fuller, S., Endress, P. L., & Johnson, J. (1978, December). The effects of cognitive and behavioral control on coping with an aversive health examination. *Journal of Human Stress*, 18–25.

Gerbert, B. (1984). Perceived likeability and competence of simulated patients: Influence on physicians' management plans. *Social Science & Medicine*, *18*, 1053–1060.

Goldstein, S., Fischer, P. M., Richards, J. W., Goldstein, A., & Shank, J. C. (1987). Smoking counseling practices of recently trained family physicians. *Journal of Family Practice*, *24*, 195–197.

Golodetz, A., Ruess, J., & Machaus, R. L. (1976). The right to know: Giving the patient his medical record. *Archives of Physical and Medical Rehabilitation*, *57*, 78–81.

Greene, M. G., Adelman, R. D., Charon, R., & Friedmann, E. (1989). Concordance between physicians and their older and younger patients in the primary care medical encounter. *The Gerontologist*, *29*, 808–813.

Greene, M., Adelman, R., Charon, R., & Hoffman, S. (1986). Ageism in the medical encounter: An exploratory study of the language and behavior of doctors with their old and young patients. *Language and Communication*, *6*, 113–124.

Greenfield, S., Kaplan, S., & Ware, J. E., Jr. (1985). Expanding patient involvement in care: Effects on patient outcomes. *Annals of Internal Medicine*, *102*, 520–528.

Greenfield, S., Kaplan, S. H., Ware, J. E., Jr., Yano, E. M., & Frank, H.J.L. (1988). Patients' participation in medical care: Effects on blood sugar control and quality of life in diabetes. *Journal of General Internal Medicine*, *3*, 448–457.

Groves, J. E. (1978). Taking care of the hateful patient. *New England Journal of Medicine*, *298*, 883–887.

Hall, J. A. (1984). *Nonverbal sex differences: Communication accuracy and expressive style*. Baltimore: Johns Hopkins University Press.

Hall, J. A. (1987). On explaining gender differences: The case of nonverbal communication. In Shaver, P., & Hendrick, C. (Eds.), *Review of Personality and Social Psychology*, *7*, Newbury Park, Calif.: Sage Publications.

Hall, J. A., & Braunwald, K. G. (1981). Gender cues in conversations. *Journal of Personality and Social Psychology*, *40*, 99–110.

Hall, J. A., & Dornan, M. C. (1988a). What patients like about their medical care and how often they are asked: A meta-analysis of the satisfaction literature. *Social Science & Medicine*, *27*, 935–939.

Hall, J. A., & Dornan, M. C. (1988b). Meta-analysis of satisfaction with medical care: Description of research domain and analysis of overall satisfaction levels. *Social Science & Medicine*, *27*, 637–644.

Hall, J. A., Epstein, A. M., DeCiantis, M. L., & McNeil, B. J. (1993). Physicians' liking for their patients: More evidence for the role of affect in medical care. *Health Psychology*, forthcoming.

Hall, J. A., Epstein, A. M., & McNeil, B. J. (1989). Multidimensionality of health status in an elderly population: Construct validity of a measurement battery. *Medical Care, 27*, S168–S177.

Hall, J. A., Feldstein, M., Fretwell, M. D., Rowe, J. W., & Epstein, A. M. (1990). Older patients' health status and satisfaction with medical care in an HMO population. *Medical Care, 28*, 261–270.

Hall, J. A., Irish, J. T., Roter, D. L., Ehrlich, C. M., Miller, L. H (1992). Gender in medical encounters: An analysis of physicians' and patients' communication behaviors. Unpublished manuscript.

Hall, J. A., Palmer, R. H., Orav, E. J., Hargraves, J. L., Wright, E. A., & Louis, T. A. (1990). Performance, quality, gender and professional role: A study of physicians and nonphysicians in sixteen ambulatory care practices. *Medical Care, 28*, 489–501.

Hall, J. A., & Roter, D. L. (1988). Physicians' knowledge and self-reported compliance promotion as predictors of performance with simulated lung disease patients. *Evaluation and the Health Professions, 11*, 306–317.

Hall, J. A., Roter, D. L., & Katz, N. R. (1987). Task versus socioemotional behaviors in physicians. *Medical Care, 25*, 399–412.

Hall, J. A., Roter, D. L., & Katz, N. R. (1988). Meta-analysis of correlates of provider behavior in medical encounters. *Medical Care, 26*, 657–675.

Hall, J. A., Roter, D. L., & Rand, C. S. (1981). Communication of affect between patient and physician. *Journal of Health and Social Behavior, 22*, 18–30.

Hall, O. (1948). The stages of a medical career. *American Journal of Sociology, 53*, 327–336.

Haug, M. R. (Ed.) (1981). *Elderly patients and their doctors.* New York: Springer Publishing.

Haug, M. R., & Lavin, B. (1981). Practitioner or patient—Who's in charge? *Journal of Health and Social Behavior, 22*, 212–229.

Haug, M., & Lavin, B. (1983). *Consumerism in medicine: Challenging physician authority.* Beverly Hills, Calif.: Sage Publications.

Haynes, R. B. (1976). A critical review of the "determinants" of patient compliance with therapeutic regimens. In Sackett, D. L., & Haynes, R. B. (Eds.), *Compliance with therapeutic regimens.* Baltimore: Johns Hopkins University Press.

Haynes, R. B., Taylor, D. W., & Sackett, D. L. (Eds.) (1981). *Compliance in health care.* 2nd ed. Baltimore: Johns Hopkins University Press.

Helfer, R. E. (1970). An objective comparison of the pediatric interviewing skills of freshman and senior medical students. *Pediatrics, 45*, 623–627.

Hemminki, E. (1975). Review of literature on the factors affecting drug prescribing. *Social Science & Medicine, 9*, 111–115.

Herman, J. M. (1985). The use of patients' preferences in family practice. *Journal of Family Practice, 20*, 153–156.

Hibbard, J. H., & Weeks, E. C. (1985). Consumer use of physician fee information. *Journal of Health and Human Resources Administration, 7*, 321–335.

Hibbard, J. H., & Weeks, E. C. (1987). Consumerism in health care: Prevalence and predictors. *Medical Care, 25*, 1019–1032.

Hilfiker, D. (1985). *Healing the wounds: A physician looks at his work.* New York: Pantheon.

Hogbin, B., & Fallowfield, L. (1989). Getting it taped: The "bad news" consultation with cancer patients. *British Journal of Hospital Medicine, 41*, 330–333.

Holder, A. R. (1970). Informed consent: Its evolution. *Journal of the American Medical Association, 214*, 1181–1182.

Hollingshead, A. B., & Redlich, F. C. (1958). *Social class and mental illness.* New York: John Wiley & Sons.

Hooper, E. M., Comstock, L. M., Goodwin, J. M., & Goodwin, J. S. (1982). Patient characteristics that influence physician behavior. *Medical Care, 20*, 630–638.

Hughs, D. (1982). Control in medical consultation: The organizing talk in a situation where co-participants have differential competence. *Sociology, 16*, 359–376.

Idler, E. L., & Kasl, S. V. (1991). Health perceptions and survival: Do global evaluations of health status really predict mortality? *Journal of Gerontology, 46*, S55–S65.

Inui, T. S., Yourtee, E. L., & Williamson, J. W. (1976). Improved outcomes in hypertension after physician tutorials: A controlled trial. *Annals of Internal Medicine, 84*, 646–651.

Jacobs, D., Carols, E., Jacobs, T., Weinstein, H., & Mann, D. (1972). Preparation for treatment of the disadvantaged patient: Effects on disposition and outcome. *American Journal of Orthopsychiatry, 42*, 666–673.

Johnson, J., Kirchoff, K., & Endress, P. (1975). Altering childrens' distress behavior during orthopedic cast removal. *Nursing Research, 24*, 404–410.

Johnson, J., & Leventhal, H. (1974). Effects of accurate expectations and behavioral instructions on reactions during a noxious medical examination. *Journal of Personality and Social Psychology, 29*, 710–718.

Jonas, H. S., & Etzel, S. (1988). Undergraduate medical education. *Journal of the American Medical Association, 260*, 1063–1071.

Kalisch, B. J. (1971). An experiment in the development of empathy in nursing students. *Nursing Research, 20*, 202–210.

Kaplan, S. H., Greenfield, S., & Ware, J. E., Jr. (1989). Assessing the effects of physician-patient interactions on the outcomes of chronic disease. *Medical Care, 27*, S110–S127.

Kelly, J. V., & Hellinger, F. J. (1986). Physician and hospital factors associated with mortality of surgical patients. *Medical Care, 24*, 785–800.

Kindelan, K., & Kent, G. (1987). Concordance between patients' information preferences and general practitioners' perceptions. *Psychology and Health, 1*, 399–409.

Klass, P. (1987). *A not entirely benign procedure: Four years as a medical student.* New York: Signet.

Kleinman, A. (1987). Explanatory models in health care relationships: A conceptual frame for research on family-based health-care activities in relation to folk and professional forms of clinical care. In Stoeckle, J. (Ed.), *Encounters between patients and doctors.* Cambridge, Mass.: MIT Press.

Koopman, C. S., Eisenthal, S., & Stoeckle, J. (1984). Ethnicity in the reported pain, emotional distress and requests of medical outpatients. *Social Science & Medicine, 6,* 487–490.

Koos, E. L. (1954). *The health of Regionville.* New York: Columbia University Press.

Korsch, B. M., Gozzi, E. K., & Francis, V. (1968). Gaps in doctor-patient communication. *Pediatrics, 42,* 855–871.

Kramer, D., Ber, R., & Moore, M. (1987). Impact of workshop on students' and physicians' rejecting behaviors in patient interview. *Journal of Medical Education, 62,* 904–910.

Krantzler, N. J. (1986). Media images of physicians and nurses in the United States. *Social Science & Medicine, 9,* 933–952.

Kulik, J. A., & Mahler, H.T.M. (1987). Effects of preoperative roommate assignment on preoperative anxiety and recovery from coronary-bypass surgery. *Health Psychology, 6,* 525–543.

Kurtz, R. A., & Chalfant, H. P. (1991). *The sociology of medicine and illness,* 2nd ed. Boston: Allyn & Bacon.

Kutner, B. (1972). Surgeons and their patients: A study in social perception. In Jaco, E. G. (Ed.), *Patients, physicians and illness.* New York: The Free Press.

Langer, E. J., & Rodin, J. (1976). The effects of choice and enhanced personal responsibility for the aged: A field experiment in an institutional setting. *Journal of Personality and Social Psychology, 34,* 191–198.

Larsson, U. S., Saljo, R., & Aronsson, K. (1987). Patient-doctor communication on smoking and drinking: Lifestyle in medical consultations. *Social Science & Medicine, 25,* 1129–1137.

Lasagna, L., Mosteller, F., von Feisinger, J. M., & Beecher, H. K. (1954). A study of the placebo response. *American Journal of Medicine, 37,* 770–779.

Lazare, A., Eisenthal, S., & Wasserman, L. (1975). The customer approach to patienthood: Attending to patient requests in a walk-in clinic. *Archives of General Psychiatry, 32,* 553–558.

Leiderman, D. B., & Grisso, J. (1985). The GOMER phenomenon. *Journal of Health and Social Behavior, 26,* 222–232.

Lewis, C. E., Lewis, M. A., Lorimer, A., & Palmer, B. B. (1977). Child-initiated care: The use of school nursing services by children in an "adult-free" system. *Pediatrics, 60,* 499–507.

Light, D. (1975). The sociological calendar: An analytic tool for fieldwork applied to medical and psychiatric training. *American Journal of Sociology, 80,* 1145–1164.

Like, R., & Zyzanski, S. J. (1987). Patient satisfaction and the clinical encounter: Social psychological determinants. *Social Science & Medicine*, *24*, 351–357.

Linn, B. S. (1982). Burn patients' evaluation of emergency department care. *Annals of Emergency Medicine*, *11*, 255–259.

Linn, L. S., Brook, R. H., Clark, V. A., Davies, A. R., Fink, A., & Kosecoff, J. (1985). Physician and patient satisfaction as factors related to the organization of internal medicine group practices. *Medical Care*, *23*, 1171–1178.

Linn, L. S., & Lewis, C. E. (1979). Attitudes toward self-care among practicing physicians. *Medical Care*, *17*, 183–190.

Lipkin, M., Jr., Quill, T. E., & Napodano, R. J. (1984). The medical interview: A curriculum for residencies in internal medicine. *Annals of Internal Medicine*, *100*, 277–284.

McKinlay, J. B. (1975). Who is really ignorant—Physician or patient? *Journal of Health and Social Behavior*, *16*, 3–11.

Mahaffy, P. R. (1965). The effects of hospitalization on children admitted for tonsillectomy and adenoidectomy. *Nursing Research*, *14*, 12–19.

Maiman, L. A., Becker, M. H., Liptak, G. S., Nazarian, L. F., & Rounds, K. A. (1988). Improving pediatricians' compliance-enhancing practices: A randomized trial. *American Journal of Diseases of Children*, *142*, 773–779.

Marshal, V. W. (1981). Physician characteristics and relationships with older patients. In Haug, M. R. (Ed.), *Elderly patients and their doctors*. New York: Springer Publishing.

Martin, D. P., Gilson, B. S., Bergner, M., Bobbitt, R. A., Pollard, W. E., Conn, J. R., & Cole, W. A. (1976). The Sickness Impact Profile: Potential use of a health status instrument for physician training. *Journal of Medical Education*, *51*, 942–947.

Maynard, C. L., Fisher, D., Passamani, E. R., & Pullum, T. (1986). Blacks in the Coronary Artery Surgery Study (CASS): Race and clinical decision making. *American Journal of Public Health*, *76*, 1446–1448.

Mechanic, D. (1974). *Politics, medicine, and social science*. New York: John Wiley & Sons.

Mechanic, D. (1978). *Medical sociology*. 2nd ed. New York: The Free Press.

Miller, R. W. (1983). Doctors, patients don't communicate. *FDA Consumer*. HHS publication no. (FDA) 83–1102.

Miller, S. M., & Mangan, C. E. (1983). Interacting effects of information and coping style in adapting to gynecologic stress: Should the doctor tell all? *Journal of Personality and Social Psychology*, *45*, 223–236.

Mills, R. T., & Krantz, D. (1979). Information choice and reactions to stress: A field experiment in a blood bank with laboratory analogue. *Journal of Personality and Social Psychology*, *37*, 608–620.

Milmoe, S., Rosenthal, R., Blane, H. T., Chafetz, M. E., & Wolf, I. (1967). The doctor's voice: Postdictor of successful referral of alcoholic patients. *Journal of Abnormal Psychology*, *72*, 78–84.

Mishler, E. G. (1984). *The discourse of medicine: Dialectics of medical interviews*. Norwood, N.J.: Ablex.

Mizrahi, T. (1986). *Getting rid of patients: Contradictions in the socialization of physicians.* New Brunswick, N.J.: Rutgers University Press.

Mumford, E., Schlesinger, H. J., & Glass, G. V. (1982). The effects of psychological intervention on recovery from surgery and heart attacks: An analysis of the literature. *American Journal of Public Health, 72,* 141–151.

Nelson, C., & McLemore, T. (1988). National Center for Health Statistics. The National Ambulatory Medical Care Survey: U.S. 1975–81, and 1985 trends. Vital and Health Statistics, series 13, no. 93, DHHS pub. no. (PHS) 88–1754. Washington, D.C.: U.S. Government Printing Office.

Nordholm, L. A. (1980). Beautiful patients are good patients: Evidence for the physical attractiveness stereotype in first impressions of patients. *Social Science & Medicine, 14A,* 81–83.

Orleans, C. T. (1985). Understanding and promoting smoking cessation: Overview and guidelines for physician intervention. *Annual Review of Medicine, 36,* 51–61.

Ornstein, S. M., Markert, G. P., Johnson, A. H., Rust, P. F., & Afrin, L. B. (1988). The effect of physician personality on laboratory test ordering for hypertensive patients. *Medical Care, 26,* 536–543.

Orth, J. E., Stiles, W. B., Scherwitz, L., Hennrikus, D., & Vallbona, C. (1987). Patient exposition and provider explanation in routine interviews and hypertensive patients' blood pressure control. *Health Psychology, 6*(1), 29–42.

Osler, W. (1904). The master-word in medicine. In *Aequanimitas, with other addresses to medical students, nurses, and practitioners of medicine.* Philadelphia: Blakiston.

Palmer, R. H., Louis, T. A., Hsu, L-N., Peterson, H. F., Rothrock, J. K., Strain, R., Thompson, M. S., & Wright, E. A. (1985). A randomized controlled trial of quality assurance in sixteen ambulatory care practices. *Medical Care, 23,* 751–770.

Palmer, R. H., & Reilly, M. C. (1979). Individual and institutional variables which may serve as indicators of quality of medical care. *Medical Care, 17,* 693–717.

Palmer, R. H., Strain, R., Maurer, J.V.W., Rothrock, J. K., & Thompson, M. S. (1984a). Quality assurance in eight adult medicine group practices. *Medical Care, 22,* 632–643.

Palmer, R. H., Strain, R., Maurer, J.V.W., & Thompson, M. S. (1984). A method for evaluating performance of ambulatory pediatric tasks. *Pediatrics, 73,* 269–277.

Parsons, T. (1951). *The social system.* Glencoe, Ill.: The Free Press.

Parsons, T. (1975). The sick role and the role of the physician reconsidered. *Milbank Memorial Fund Quarterly, 53,* 257–278.

Pascoe, G. C. (1983). Patient satisfaction in primary health care: A literature review and analysis. *Evaluation and Program Planning, 6,* 185–210.

Pendleton, D. A., & Bochner, S. (1980). The communication of medical information in general practice consultations as a function of patients' social class. *Social Science & Medicine, 14A,* 669–673.

Pendleton, L., & House, W. C. (1984). Preferences for treatment approaches in medical care: College students versus diabetic outpatients. *Medical Care, 22*, 644–646.

Pickering, G. (1979). Therapeutics: Art or science? *Journal of the American Medical Association, 242*, 649–653.

Pratt, L., Seligmann, A., & Reader, G. (1957). Physicians' views on the level of medical information among patients. *American Journal of Public Health, 47*, 1277–1283.

President's Commission for the Study of Ethical Problems in Medicine and Biomedical and Behavioral Research. (1982). *Making health care decisions: The ethical and legal implications of informed consent in the patient-practitioner relationship*. Vol. 1. Washington, D.C.: U.S. Government Printing Office.

Price, J. H., Desmond, S. M., Snyder, F. F., & Kimmel, S. R. (1988). Perceptions of family practice residents regarding health care and poor patients. *Journal of Family Practice, 27*, 615–621.

Quill, T. E. (1983). Partnerships in patient care: A contractual approach. *Annals of Internal Medicine, 98*, 228–234.

Quine, L., & Pahl, J. (1986). First diagnosis of severe mental handicap: Characteristics of unsatisfactory encounters between doctors and parents. *Social Science & Medicine, 22*, 53–62.

Quint, J. (1972). Institutionalized practices of information control. In Freidson, E., & Lorber, J. (Eds.), *Medical men and their work: A sociological reader*. Chicago: Aldine Atherton.

Rabin, D. L., & Bush, P. J. (1975). Who's using medicines? *Journal of Community Health, 1*, 106–117.

Reader, G. S., Pratt, L., & Mudd, M. C. (1957). What do patients expect from their doctors? *Modern Hospital, 89*, 88–91.

Reeder, L. G. (1972). The patient-client as a consumer: Some observations on the changing professional-client relationship. *Journal of Health and Social Behavior, 13*, 406–412.

Rhee, S. (1977). Relative importance of physicians' personal and situational characteristics for the quality of patient care. *Journal of Health and Social Behavior, 18*, 10–15.

Rhee, S. O. (1983). Organizational determinants of medical care quality: A review of the literature. In Luke, R. D., Krueger, J. C., & Modrow, R. E. (Eds.), *Organization and change in health care quality assurance*. Rockville, Md.: Aspen.

Robertson, W. O. (1985). *Medical malpractice: A preventive approach*. Seattle: University of Washington Press.

Rodin, J., & Langer, E. J. (1977). Long-term effects of a control-relevant intervention with the institutionalized aged. *Journal of Personality and Social Psychology, 35*, 897–902.

Rogoff, N. (1957). The decision to study medicine. In Merton, R. K., Reader, G. G., & Kendall, P. L. (Eds.), *The student-physician*. Cambridge, Mass.: Harvard University Press.

Rosengren, W. R. (1980). *Sociology of medicine: Diversity, conflict and change.* New York: Harper & Row.

Rosenthal, R., Hall, J. A., DiMatteo, M. R., Rogers, P. L., & Archer, D. (1979). *Sensitivity to nonverbal communication: The PONS test.* Baltimore: Johns Hopkins University Press.

Rosenthal, R., Vannicelli, M., & Blanck, P. (1984). Speaking to and about patients: Predicting therapists' tone of voice. *Journal of Consulting and Clinical Psychology, 52,* 679–686.

Ross, C. R., & Duff, R. S. (1982). Returning to the doctor: The effects of client characteristics, type of practice, and experiences with care. *Journal of Health and Social Behavior, 23,* 119–131.

Rost, K., & Roter, D. (1987). Predictors of recall of medication regimens and recommendations for lifestyle change in elderly patients. *The Gerontologist, 27,* 510–515.

Roter, D. (1977). Patient participation in the patient-provider interaction: The effects of patient question asking on the quality of interaction, satisfaction, and compliance. *Health Education Monographs, 5,* 281–315.

Roter, D. L. (1984). Patient question asking in physician-patient interaction. *Health Psychology, 3,* 395–409.

Roter, D. (1991). Elderly patient-physician communication: A descriptive study of content and affect during the medical encounter. *Advances in Health Education, 3,* 15–23.

Roter, D. L., & Hall, J. A. (1987). Physicians' interviewing styles and medical information obtained from patients. *Journal of General Internal Medicine, 2,* 325–329.

Roter, D. L., Hall, J. A., & Katz, N. R. (1987). Relations between physicians' behaviors and analogue patients' satisfaction, recall, and impressions. *Medical Care, 25,* 437–451.

Roter, D. L., Hall, J. A., & Katz, N. R. (1988). Patient-physician communication: A descriptive summary of the literature. *Patient Education and Counseling, 12,* 99–119.

Roter, D., Lipkin, M., Jr., & Korsgaard, A. (1991). Sex differences in patients' and physicians' communication during primary care medical visits. *Medical Care, 29,* 1083–1093.

Roth, J. A. (1963). Information and the control of treatment in tuberculosis hospitals. In Freidson, E., *The hospital in modern society.* London: The Free Press of Glencoe.

Rubenstein, L. Z., Schairer, C., Wieland, G. D., & Kane, R. (1984). Systematic biases in functional status assessment of elderly adults: Effects of different data sources. *Journal of Gerontology, 39,* 686–691.

Russell, N. K., & Roter, D. L. (1992). Discussion of lifestyle topics with chronic disease patients in primary care medical visits. *American Journal of Public Health,* forthcoming.

Sanazaro, P. J., & Worth, R. M. (1985). Measuring clinical performance of individual internists in office and hospital practice. *Medical Care, 23,* 1097–1114.

Sarason, B. R., Sarason, I. G., Hacker, T. A., & Basham, R. B. (1985). Concomitants of social support: Social skills, physical attractiveness, and gender. *Journal of Personality and Social Psychology*, *49*, 469–480.

Schmitt, F. E., & Woolridge, P. J. (1973). Psychological preparation of surgical patients. *Nursing Research*, *22*, 108–116.

Scully, D. (1980). *Men who control women's health: The miseducation of obstetrician-gynecologists*. Boston: Houghton Mifflin.

Shapiro, R. S., Simpson, D. E., & Lawrence, S. L. (1989). A survey of sued and nonsued physicians and suing patients. *Archives of Internal Medicine*, *149*, 2190–2196.

Shenkin, B., & Warner, D. (1973). Giving the patient his medical record: A proposal to improve the system. *New England Journal of Medicine*, *289*, 688–691.

Shorter, E. (1985). *Bedside manners*. New York: Simon and Schuster.

Skipper, J. K., Tagliacozzo, D. L., & Mauksch, H. O. (1964). Some possible consequences of limited communication between patients and hospital functionaries. *Journal of Health and Human Behavior*, *6*, 34.

Smith, R. C., & Zimny, G. H. (1988). Physicians' emotional reactions to patients. *Psychosomatics*, *29*, 392–397.

Speedling, E. J., & Rose, D. N. (1985). Building an effective doctor-patient relationship: From patient satisfaction to patient participation. *Social Science & Medicine*, *21*, 115–120.

Steptoe, A., Sutcliffe, I., Allen, B., & Coombes, C. (1991). Satisfaction with communication, medical knowledge, and coping style in patients with metastatic cancer. *Social Science & Medicine*, *32*, 627–632.

Stevens, D. P., & MacKay, C. R. (1977). What happens when hospitalized patients see their records? *Annals of Internal Medicine*, *86*, 474–477.

Stewart, M. (1983). Patient characteristics which are related to the doctor-patient interaction. *Family Practice*, *1*, 30–35.

Stewart, M. (1984). What is a successful doctor-patient interview? A study of interactions and outcomes. *Social Science & Medicine*, *19*, 167–175.

Stimson, G. V. (1974). Obeying doctor's orders: A view from the other side. *Social Science & Medicine*, *8*, 97–104.

Stimson, G. V. & Webb, B. (1975). *Going to see the doctor: The consultation process in general practice*. London: Routledge & Kegan Paul.

Stoeckle, J. D., & Barsky, A. (1981). Attributions: Uses of social science knowledge in doctoring in primary care. In Eisenberg, L., & Kleinman, A. (Eds.), *The relevance of social science for medicine*. Boston: D. Reidel.

Stolley, P. D., Becker, M. H., Lasagna, L., McEvilla, J. D., & Sloane, L. M. (1972). The relationship between physician characteristics and prescribing appropriateness. *Medical Care*, *10*, 17–28.

Strull, W. M., Lo, B., & Charles, G. (1984). Do patients want to participate in medical decision making? *Journal of the American Medical Association*, *252*, 2990–2994.

Suchman, A. L., & Matthews, D. A. (1988). What makes the patient-doctor relationship therapeutic?: Exploring the connexional dimension of medical care. *Annals of Internal Medicine, 108*, 125–130.

Svarstad, B. L. (1974). *The doctor-patient encounter: An observational study of communication and outcome.* Doctoral dissertation, University of Wisconsin, Madison.

Szasz, P. S., & Hollender, M. H. (1956). A contribution to the philosophy of medicine: The basic model of the doctor-patient relationship. *Archives of Internal Medicine, 97*, 585–592.

Tagliacozzo, D. L., & Mauksch, H. O. (1972). The patient's view of the patient role. In Jaco, E. G. (Ed.), *Patients, physicians and illness.* New York: The Free Press.

Thomas, K. B. (1978). The consultation and the therapeutic illusion. *British Medical Journal, 1*, 1327–1328.

Tobin, J. N., Wassertheil-Smoller, S., Wexler, J. P., Steingart, R. M., Budner, N., Lense, L., & Wachspress, J. (1987). Sex bias in considering coronary bypass surgery. *Annals of Internal Medicine, 107*, 19–25.

Tuckett, D., Boulton, M., Olson, C., & Williams, A. (1985). *Meetings between experts.* New York: Tavistock Publications.

Tudor, C. (1988). Career plans and debt levels of graduating U.S. medical students, 1981–1986. *Journal of Medical Education, 63*, 271–275.

U.S. Department of Health and Human Services. (1982). *The health consequences of smoking: Cancer.* Washington, D.C.: U.S. Government Printing Office.

Vannicelli, M., & Blanck, P. (1984). Speaking to and about patients: Predicting therapists' tone of voice. *Journal of Consulting and Clinical Psychology, 52*, 679–686.

Verbrugge, L. M., & Steiner, R. P. (1981). Physician treatment of men and women patients: Sex bias or appropriate care? *Medical Care, 19*, 609–632.

Vertinsky, I. B., Thompson, W. A., & Uyeno, D. (1974). Measuring consumer desire for participation in clinical decision making. *Health Services Research, 9*, 121–134.

Waitzkin, H. (1985). Information giving in medical care. *Journal of Health and Social Behavior, 26*, 81–101.

Waitzkin, H., & Waterman, B. (1974). *The exploitation of illness in capitalist society.* New York: Bobbs-Merrill.

Wallen, J., Waitzkin, H., & Stoeckle, J. D. (1979). Physician stereotypes about female health and illness. *Women & Health, 4*, 135–146.

Wang, V., Terry, P., Flynn, B., Williamson, J., Green, L., & Faden, R. (1979). Evaluation of continuing medical education for chronic obstructive pulmonary diseases. *Journal of Medical Education, 54*, 803–811.

Wartman, S. A., Morlock, L. L., Malitz, F. E., & Palm, E. (1981). Do prescriptions adversely affect doctor-patient interactions? *American Journal of Public Health, 71*, 1358–1361.

Wasserman, R. C., Inui, T. S., Barriatua, R. D., Carter, W. B., & Lippincott, P. (1983). Responsiveness to maternal concern in preventive child health visits: An analysis of clinician-parent interactions. *Developmental and Behavioral Pediatrics, 4*, 171–176.

Wasserman, R. C., Inui, T. S., Barriatua, R. D., Carter, W. B., & Lippincott, P. (1984). Pediatric clinicians' support for parents makes a difference: An outcome-based analysis of clinician-parent interaction. *Pediatrics, 74*, 1047–1053.

Weisman, C. S., & Teitelbaum, M. A. (1989). Women and health care communication. *Patient Education and Counseling, 13*, 183–199.

West, P. (1976). The physician and the management of childhood epilepsy. In Wadsworth, D. (Ed.), *Studies in everyday medical life*. Oxford: Martin Robertson.

White, K. L. (1988). *The task of medicine: Dialogue at Wickenburg*. Menlo Park, Calif.: Henry J. Kaiser Family Foundation.

Willson, P., & McNamara, J. R. (1982). How perceptions of a simulated physician-patient interaction influence intended satisfaction and compliance. *Social Science & Medicine, 16*, 1699–1703.

Wintrobe, M. M., Thorn, G. W., Adams, R. D., Bennett, I. L., Jr., Braunwald, E., Isselbacher, K. J., & Petersdorf, R. G. (Eds.) (1970). *Harrison's principles of internal medicine*. New York: McGraw-Hill.

Wu, A. W., Folkman, S., McPhee, S. J., & Lo, B. (1991). Do house officers learn from their mistakes? *Journal of the American Medical Association, 265*, 2089–2094.

Yager, J., & Linn, L. S. (1981). Physician-patient agreement about depression: Notation in medical records. *General Hospital Psychiatry, 3*, 271–276.

Zborowski, M. (1952). Cultural components in responses to pain. *Journal of Social Issues, 4*, 16–30.

Zola, I. K. (1963). Problems of communication, diagnosis, and patient care: The interplay of patient, physician and clinic organization. *Journal of Medical Education, 38*, 829–838.

Zola, I. K. (1966). Culture and symptoms: An analysis of patients' presenting complaints. *American Sociological Review, 31*, 615–630.

Zuckerman, M., & Driver, R. E. (1985). Telling lies: Verbal and nonverbal correlates of deception. In Siegman, A. W., & Feldstein, S. (Eds.), *Multichannel integrations of nonverbal behavior*. Hillsdale, N.J.: Erlbaum.

Subject Index

Age: attitudes related to patient's, 40–42; behavior related to physician's or patient's, 40–42, 53, 122, 137, 162

Anger, 34, 41, 44, 51, 81, 84, 85, 138, 141, 148. *See also* Negative talk

Anxiety, 3, 7, 13, 14, 17, 26, 43, 81, 84, 85, 86, 91, 98, 100, 101, 104, 138, 148, 151, 152–154, 157, 159, 167. *See also* Negative talk

Appearance, 40, 50, 51, 52, 53

Attributions, 7, 13–14, 16, 49, 105, 136–137, 141, 146, 148

Baby talk, 41

Back channel responses, 44, 84

Bills, payment of, 15

Biomedical model, 23, 126, 162

Compliance, 12–13, 15, 22, 23, 25, 70, 98, 126, 131, 132, 138, 139–146, 148, 151, 156, 159–161. *See also* Prescriptions

Consumerism: as model of doctor-patient relationship, 13, 24, 27–32, 34, 65, 66, 67; in society, 12, 28, 132

Control, 24–25, 31, 33–34, 81, 83, 89, 100, 135, 142, 146, 147, 153, 154–156, 158, 167. *See also* Locus of control

Cost-consciousness, 28–29

Courtesy, 16, 42

Default, 24–25, 33–34

Diagnosis, 5, 12, 96, 97, 102, 111, 132, 148, 158, 160, 163, 167, 173; difficulty of making, 10–11, 113, 119, 127. *See also* Test ordering

"Doctor-centered" communication, 89–91

Dominance, 84, 89, 136, 140, 147

Drugs. *See* Prescriptions

Education, models of, 12. *See also* Teacher, physician as

Emotional distress, 10, 11, 14, 52, 112, 126, 138–139, 162, 164

Author Index

About the Authors

DEBRA L. ROTER is an Associate Professor at Johns Hopkins University where she teaches in the School of Hygiene and Public Health.

JUDITH A. HALL is a Professor of Psychology at Northeastern University.